AF601565

Innovations in Biochemical Techniques

The Editors

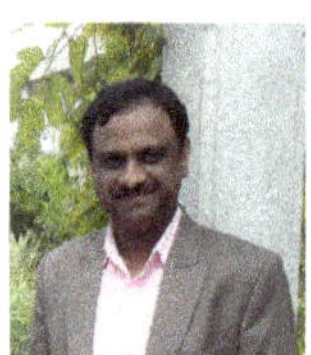

Dr. Sadashiv S. O. [M. Sc., M. Phil., Ph. D.,] presently is serving as an Assistant Professor, in the Department of Food Technology, Davangere University, Davanagere, Karnataka. He has completed M. Phil and Ph.D. in Microbiology from Karnatak University, Dharwad, Karnataka, India. He has published various research articles in national and international peer reviewed journals and 6 book chapters, 2 Books/Monographs, and edited 4 books. He has secured two times Young Scientists Award, one Gold Medal award for the research contributions in the field of Veterinary Microbiology from various academic organizations, and also received Appreciation Award from Zoological Society of India (ZSI). He has participated and presented research paper in many conferences/ seminar/ workshop/ trainings at national and international levels. His thrust areas of research are Veterinary Microbiology, Dairy Microbiology, Environmental Microbiology and Food Technology.

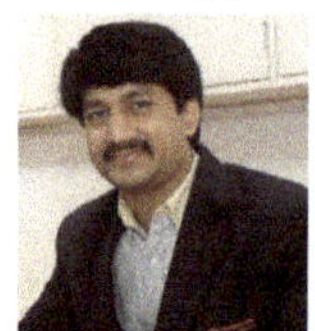

Dr. Sharangouda J. Patil [M.Sc.,B.Ed., Ph.D., PDF] completed his Masters (II Rank) in Zoology, subsequently he completed his Doctorate from Gulbarga University, Gulbarga during 2007. Thereafter he has completed post-doctoral fellowship (PDF) in World Bank funded project in ICAR reputed National Institute of Animal Nutrition and Physiology, Bangalore. For his post-doctoral research Dr. Patil opted to work on livestock extension research extensively. His work involved field research as well as lab research. With his skills and techniques he was very useful for farmers. He has made major contributions in outreach programs of the institute for transfer of technology from lab to land. He also worked in software industry as a Subject Matter Expert of Zoology to develop a E-contents for UG and PG level of all the Karnataka state universities in 2016. During his teaching and research career, he has published more than 56 research articles, 5 book chapters, 5 technical bulletins and several other technical articles in National and International peer reviewed journals. Currently he is working as Associate Professor in School of Sciences, Department of Life Sciences, Garden City University, Bangalore from the 2017 onwards and has around 12 year teaching and research experience in the field of Zoology, Genetics, Biotechnology and Microbiology.

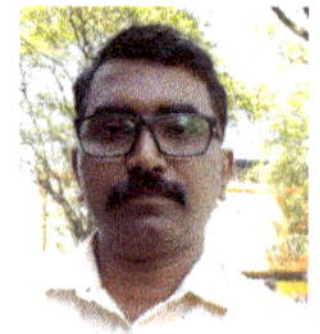

Dr. Vishwanatha T. [M. Sc., M. Phil., Ph.D.,] is a focused microbiologist, Assistant Professor in Maharani's Science College for Women, Bangalore. He has an outstanding career with 14 years of teaching and research experience. He has obtained his Master of Philosophy and Doctor of Philosophy from Gulbarga University, Karnataka. During his research has explored bacteriophage as a potential antimicrobial agent against the MDR strains of Staphylococcus aureus. Till now he has 27 publications and he secured several awards for presenting his papers at national and international level seminar and conferences. He has underwent many faculty development program and refresher courses. His main area of research is phage therapy.

Innovations in Biochemical Techniques

Editors

Dr. Sadashiv S.O.
Dr. Sharangouda J. Patil
Dr. Vishwanatha T.

2020

Daya Publishing House®

A Division of

Astral International Pvt. Ltd.

New Delhi – 110 002

ISBN: 9789390371624 (Int Edition)

Published by : **Daya Publishing House®**
A Division of
Astral International Pvt. Ltd.
– ISO 9001:2015 Certified Company –
4736/23, Ansari Road, Darya Ganj
New Delhi-110 002
Ph. 011-43549197, 23278134
E-mail: info@astralint.com
Website: www.astralint.com

Preface

The current technological boom has put forth a variety of research techniques, methods, protocols being used in life science teaching and research in higher education. There is now more than ever a great deal of interaction between the chemical, physical and biological sciences. The biologist today depends on recent advances in life science study in the aspects of physiology, biochemistry, biotechnology, microbiology, genetics, pharmacology, toxicology, environmental biology of living organisms, particularly at the molecular level studies. A several technologies have been developed over the years to address the challenges of different disciplines of life science. There is a need for a thorough understanding of the basic principles, theories and methods were involved in the outcome of research findings and various parameters like, chemical, physical and biological studies in that required to develop newer approach and strategies for future researchers. This book is an endeavor for young researchers, budding scientists, academicians and industry people.

The Innovations in Biochemical Techniques book include twelve chapters that amalgamate from the basic to advanced investigations that hold the modern impetus in research and development. The book deals with various aspects of research work having principles, theories, methods, protocols, concepts, techniques and applications with wide range experimental outcomes in *in-vitro* and *in-vivo* studies.

All the chapters have been organized from the basic to applied research innovations with appropriate illustrations to make them comprehensive. The book will be useful for young researchers in the field of biological science and other allied branch of sciences and it will be use it as research tools & techniques currently in practice. The book fine tunes the methods behind the various experiments, using different instruments that illustrate the seed of prospective rationale in research students. All twelve chapters emphasize a well-defined methodology that describes the research innovations and their applications in different fields of life science, illuminating the young minds of various level knocking on the door or innovative research.

A unique facet of this book is its broad coverage of subjects that incorporates fundamental concepts of biochemical assays, histopathology, micrometry, gravimetry, cell culture, cell lines, toxicity, radio-immuno assays, behavioral, fermentation, bioprocess, phytochemistry, synthesis of nanoparticles, biofuel, biopesticide, Food Borne Diseases, and also advocates the important applications of modern molecular and genetic engineering tools that lay the basis for state-of the-art of research in the present era of oncology, stem cell research, metagenomics, metaproteomics, metabolomics, genomic engineering, nanobionics, molecular markers, data science and spectroscopy.

The present aspects of biochemistry, biotechnology, genetics and microbiology will provide readers with comprehensive insight into the dynamics of the core commercial application to industrial research and development, a sanguine component that has been missing in contemporary books related to biological science. The book can also help to researchers by laying down the inventory of research methods and their various approach that could be put to practice to further investigation.

Dr. Sadashiv S. O.

Dr. Sharangouda J. Patil

Dr. Vishwanatha T.

Contents

Innovations in Biochemical Techniques (2020) : Page no. 1-7
ASTRAL INTERNATIONAL (P) LTD., New Delhi - 110002

Chapter 1

In Vitro Analysis of Biocompatibility of Graphene Oxide Nanoparticles

Nila Nandhini Muthu Kumar,[a] *Nikhil K. Kothurkar,*[b] *L. Surendran*[c]

Department of Electronics & Communication Engineering,[a] *Department of Chemical Engineering & Materials Science* [b], *Amrita School of Engineering, Coimbatore, Amrita Vishwa Vidyapeetham, India, 641112. E-mail: k_nikhil@cb.amrita.edu PG and Research Department of Biotechnology* [c], *Kongunadu Arts and Science College, Coimbatore-641029.*

Abstract

Introduction: Nowadays the nanoparticle based therapies becoming familiar and emerging among the other therapeutic methods in the field of physics, chemistry and biomedical sciences. Since from the ancient history the metal ion based treatments was existed *i.e.* silver ions was used in biological applications. The present research investigated *in-vitro* the biocompatibility of the graphene oxideNPs nanoparticles on 3T3 mouse fibroblasts cell lines.

Materials and Methods: To check the biocompatible property of graphene oxide NPs, we have employed few *in-vitro* cytological techniques. At first the synthesized graphene oxide was preliminary characterized by using UV-Visible spectrophotometer and peak was absorbed at 310nm wavelength. Then the graphene oxide NPs was forwarded to check biocompatibility on 3T3 mouse fibroblasts cell lines using MTT cytotoxicity assay. Afterwards the graphene oxide NPs was analysed to Genotoxicity over the DNA fragmentation and comet assay.

Results: From the results, we ensured that, the graphene oxide NPs is not having any cytotoxic effects on 3T3 mouse fibroblasts cell lines, proved over the absorbance readings of MTT. Also there was no Genotoxicity recorded throughout the concentration from 60μg up to 850μg/mL on comet assay.

Discussion: So finally the graphene oxide NPs does not suspected at any concentrations as toxic and we confirmed that, the graphene oxide NPs can be applicable to biological application at safer level and future investigations may proves the biocompatible property of graphene oxide NPs.

Keywords: *Graphene oxide NPs, MTT assay, Biocompatibility, DNA fragmentation, Comet assay*

Introduction

Nowadays the nanoparticle based therapies becoming familiar and emerging among the other therapeutic methods in the field of physics, chemistry and biomedical sciences. Since from the ancient history the metal ion based treatments was existed *i.e.* silver ions was used in biological applications (Graves J. *et al.*, 2015). The biological assays were employed to study the drug or nanoparticles for its biocompatibility. Most of the scientists have been performed MTT cytotoxicity assay for checking the nanoparticle and other king on chemical compounds (Moradhaseli S *et al.*, 2013). Because once a molecules or NPs enters into the body, it may react with any king of biomolecules such as DNA, proteins, enzymes and lipids according to the binding nature (Na K *et al.*, 2000) Especially if the drug molecule is a metal ion, definitely we must check the biocompatibility of them and also compared with other drug molecules, the NPs are highly accumulated into the body tissues. But most of the NPs did not excrete properly and scientists have been reported that they caused more problems inside the cell due to the size. So that nanoparticles are checked for its biocompatibility (Win KY *et al.*, 2005). Also in biotechnology nowadays the graphene oxide carbon NPs becoming familiar on therapies than the others, especially the antibacterial activity and biocompatibility. Already the graphene oxide NPs has approved for the filtration process in the water purifier and now became a biocompatible one among other NPs. The present research investigated *in-vitro* the biocompatibility of the graphene oxide NPs nanoparticles on 3T3 mouse fibroblasts cell lines (Sahoo SK *et al.*, 2005).

Materials and Methods

Synthesis of Graphene Oxide

The Graphene oxide nanoparticle was synthesized and tested for the biocompatibility on cell lines.

Characterization of graphene oxide (Nica IC, Stan MS, Popa M, *et al.*, 2017)

The synthesized graphene oxide was preliminarily characterized by using UV-Visible spectrophotometer at full scan mode, which scans the graphene oxide from 200 to 800nm wavelength. Here 1mL of synthesized graphene oxide suspension was used for the characterization.

Culture of Mouse Fibroblast Cell lines (Carlisle *et al.*, 2000; Lieber *et al.*, 1976)

The Mouse fibroblasts cell line was obtained from NCCS pune. Then the culture was checked for contamination and viability. Afterwards the culture was fed with DMEM (Dulbecco's minimal essential medium, Hi-media labs) medium with medium glucose and 10% FBS (Fetal bovine serum, Hi-media) was added and maintained at 37 degree Celsius with 5% CO_2.

Preparations of graphene oxide (Rajesh Kumar S, Rout B, *et al.*, 2018)

The graphene oxide was prepared at different concentration to check the biocompatibility on mouse fibroblast cell lines. The graphene oxide was prepared as five different concentrations as from 60µg/mL, 120µg/mL, 250µg/mL, 550µg/mL and up to 850µg/mL.

MTT Cytotoxicity Assay *(Mossman T, 1983)*

MTT cell proliferation and viability assay is a safe, sensitive, in vitro based assay for evaluate the cell proliferation or, lead to apoptosis or necrosis, a reduction in the cell population. The mouse fibroblast Cells were cultured in flat-bottomed, 96-well tissue culture plates and the Suspension of Graphene oxide was added at concentration (6, 12, 25, 55, and 85μL respectively). The added suspensions containing 60μg/6μL, 120μg/12μL, 250μg/25μL, 550μg/55μL, 850μg/85μL.The mouse fibroblasts were treated as per experimental design and incubation times are optimized for each cell type and system. The tetrazolium compound MTT (3-[4, 5-dimethylthiazol-2-yl]-2, 5-diphenyltetrazolium bromide) was added to the wells and then the mouse fibroblasts were incubated 37 degree Celsius. MTT is reduced by metabolically active mouse fibroblasts cells to insoluble purple Formazan dye crystals. Afterwards a solvent was added to solubilizing the crystals, so the absorbance was read using micro plate reader (Bio-Rad, UK). The cells were read directly into the wells and the optimal wavelength for absorbance is 570 nm, the data was evaluated by plotting concentration of graphene oxide versus absorbance, allowing quantitation of changes in cell proliferation. The change of tetrazolium reduction is proportional to the rate of cell proliferation.

Comet Assay for Checking of Genotoxicity *(Singh et al., 1988)*

The comet assay was performed to graphene oxide on mouse fibroblast cell for checking the Genotoxicity. The mouse fibroblast cells were treated with low and high doses of graphene oxide and incubated for 24hrs at 37 degree Celsius with 5% CO2. Then the cells were coved as sandwich with low melting and high melting agarose. Then it was stained with fluorescent dye propidium iodide (a DNA binding fluorescent dye) and the sandwich was placed on electrophoresis apparatus to find the elevation of DNA from the cell. The result was visualized using fluorescent microscope, where normal cell appears red colour round dot like structure, but the DNA damaged cell appears comet like structure.

Results and Discussions

Synthesis and Characterization of Graphene Oxide

The graphene oxide nanoparticles synthesized and gave satisfied results. The synthesized graphene oxide was characterized by using the UV-Visible spectrophotometer. The synthesis was confirmed by the peak reading at 310nm wave length (Nica IC, Stan MS, Popa M, *et al.*, 2017).So finally the synthesized graphene oxide NP was clear and gave a peak values at 310nm withabsorbance value of 0.5 to 0.6A, which denotes the solution of graphene oxide nanoparticle not containing any crosscontamination.

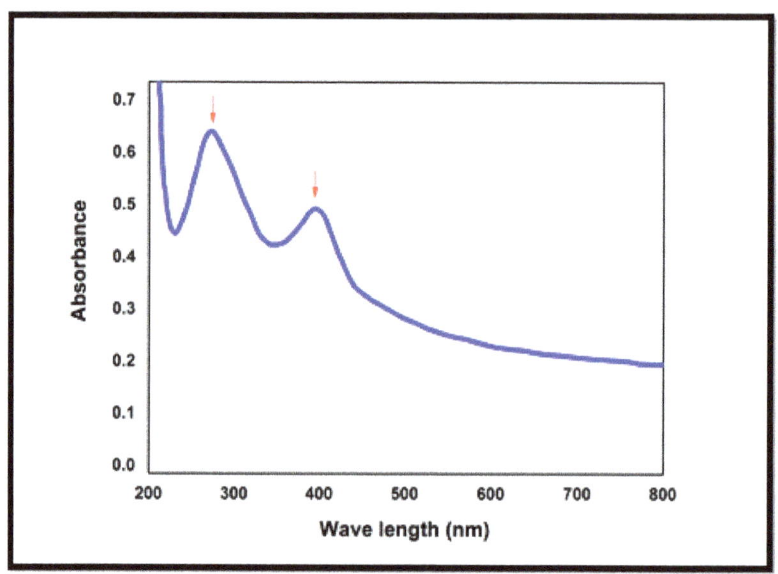

Fig 1: Characterization of graphene oxide using UV-Visible spectrophotometer

MTT Cytotoxicity Assay

The MTT assay was performed to check the biocompatibility of graphene oxide on mouse fibroblasts cells. The results obtained from the MTT assay, the treatment of graphene oxide with mouse fibroblast cells and we observed satisfied live cell viability percentage throughout the doses from 60µg to 850µg (Lu X *et al.*, 2011). compared with control (Untreated) 98% all those concentrations does not gave considerable cell death on the population (Zakrzewska KE *et al.*, 2015).

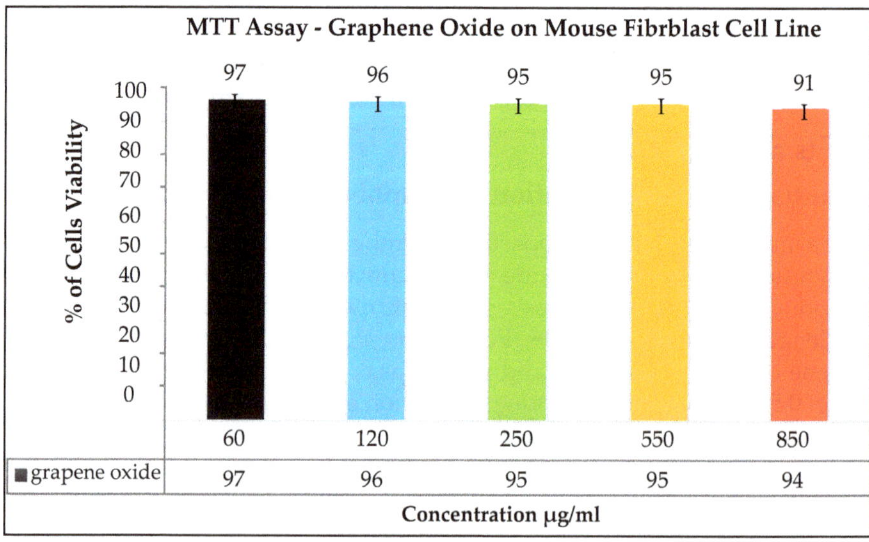

	60	120	250	550	850
■ grapene oxide	97	96	95	95	94

Graph.1: MTT assay for graphene oxide NPs on 3T3-Mouse fibroblast cells.

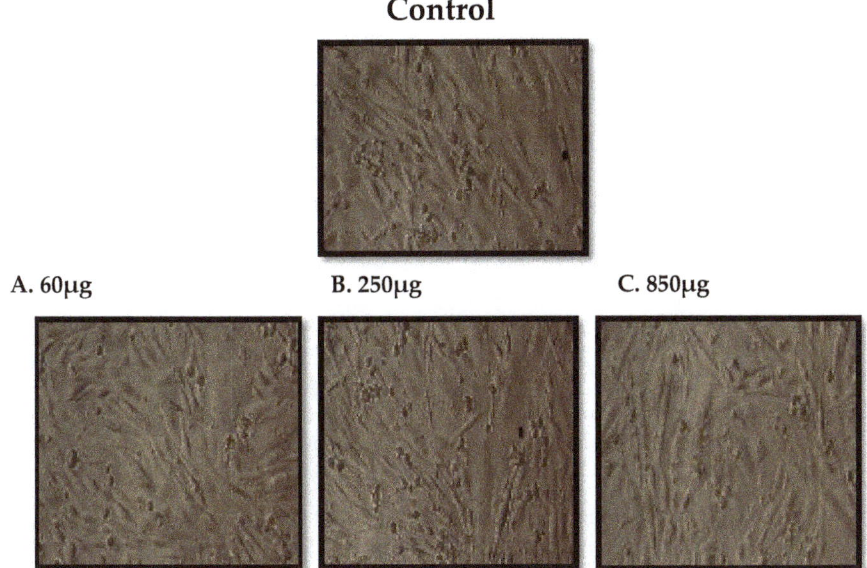

Fig 2: Inverted phase contrast microscopic analysis of graphene oxide NPs on 3T3-Mouse fibroblast cells at different concentrations.

Comet Assay for Checking of Genotoxicity

The comet assay was performed to graphene oxide on 3T3-mouse fibroblast cell for checking of Genotoxicity and DNA fragmentation. From the results we obtained in the comet assay, as like MTT assay this also did not produce any cellular damage and DNA fragmentation, during the treatment of graphene oxide NPs at low to high doses. All the slides were visualized under fluorescent microscopy with aid propidium iodide (A DNA binding fluorescent dye). There was no comet like structures were observed at any concentration (Bengtson S *et al.,* 2016).

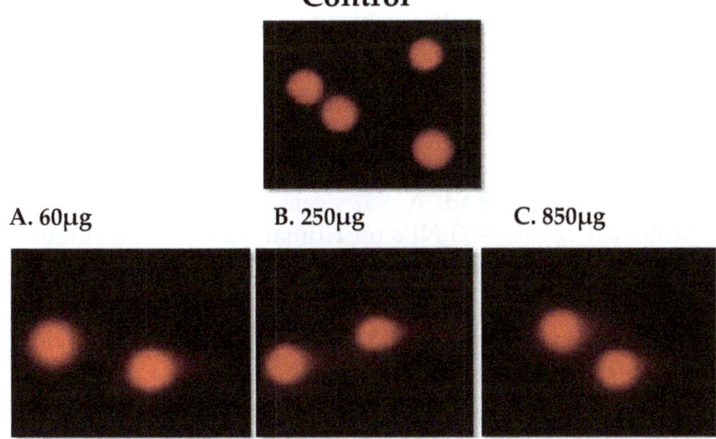

Fig 3: Fluorescent microscopic images of comet assay of graphene oxide NPs on 3T3-Mouse fibroblast cells at different concentrations.

Conclusion

From the discussion, we ensured that, the graphene oxide NPs is not having any cytotoxic effects on 3T3 mouse fibroblasts cell lines, proved over the absorbance readings of MTT. Also there was no Genotoxicity recorded throughout the concentration from 60µg up to 850µg/mL on comet assay. So finally the graphene oxide NPs does not suspected at any concentrations as toxic and we confirmed that, the graphene oxide NPs can be applicable to biological application at safer level and future investigations may proves the biocompatible property of graphene oxide NPs.

References

Ahoo SK, Ma W, Labhasetwar V. Efficacy of transferrin-conjugated paclitaxel loaded nanoparticles in a murine model of prostate cancer. *Int. J. Cancer*. 2004; 112: 335–40.

Bengtson S, Kling K, Madsen AM, *et al*. No cytotoxicity or genotoxicity of graphene and graphene oxide in murine lung epithelial FE1 cells *in vitro*. *Environmental and Molecular Mutagenesis*. 2016;57(6):469-482. doi:10.1002/em.22017.

Carlisle, D.L., Pritchard, D.E., Singh, J., Owens, B.M., Blankenship, L.J., Orenstein, J.M., Patierno, S.R., 2000. Apoptosis and P53 induction in human lung fibroblastsexposed to chromium (VI): effect of ascorbate and tocopherol. *Toxicol. Sci.* 55, 60-68.

Graves J., Jr., Tajkarimi M., Cunningham Q., Campbell A., Nonga H., Harrison S., E Barrick J. Rapid evolution of silver nanoparticle resistance in *Escherichia coli*. *Front. Genet*. 2015;6:42.

Jackson P, Pedersen LM, Kyjovska ZO, Jacobsen NR, Saber AT, Hougaard KS, Vogel U, Wallin H. 2013. Validation of freezing tissues and cells for analysis of DNA strand break levels by comet assay. *Mutagenesis* 28:699–707.

Lieber, M., Smith, B., Szakal, A., Nelson-Rees, W., Todaro, G., 1976. A continuoustumor-cell line from a human lung carcinoma with properties of type II alveolarepithelial cells. *Int. J. Cancer*.17, 62-70.

Lu X, Qian J, Zhou H, Gan Q, Tang W, Lu J, *et al*. *In vitro* cytotoxicity and induction of apoptosis by silica nanoparticles in human HepG2 hepatoma cells. *Int J Nanomedicine*. 2011; 6.

Moradhaseli S, Zare Mirakabadi A, Sarzaeem A, Kamalzadeh M, Haji Hosseini R. Cytotoxicity of ICD-85 NPs on Human Cervical Carcinoma HeLa Cells through Caspase-8 Mediated Pathway. *Iranian Journal of Pharmaceutical Research : IJPR*. 2013;12(1):155-163.

Mossman T, 1983. Rapid colorimetric assay for cellular growth and survival: application to proliferation and cytotoxicity assays. *J Immunol Meth*. 65, 55-63.

Muzyka R, Drewniak S, Pustelny T, Chrubasik M, Gryglewicz G. Characterization of Graphite Oxide and Reduced Graphene Oxide Obtained from Different

Graphite Precursors and Oxidized by Different Methods Using Raman Spectroscopy. *Materials.* 2018; 11 (7):1050.

Na K, Park KH, Kim SW, Bae YH. Self-assembled hydrogel nanoparticles from curdlan derivatives: characterization, anti-cancer drug release and interaction with a hepatoma cell line (HepG2) *J. Control. Release.* 2000; 69: 225–36.

Nica IC, Stan MS, Popa M, *et al.* Development and Biocompatibility Evaluation of Photocatalytic TiO_2/Reduced Graphene Oxide-Based Nanoparticles Designed for Self-Cleaning Purposes. *Nanomaterials.* 2017;7(9):279.

Rajesh Kumar S, Rout B, *et al.* The Preparation of Graphene Oxide-Silver Nanocomposites: The Effect of Silver Loads on Gram-Positive and Gram-Negative Antibacterial Activities. *Nanomaterials.* 2018;8(3):163. doi:10.3390/nano8030163.

Singh N P, McCoy M T, Tice R R and Schneider E L., 1988. A simple technique for quantification of low level DNA damage in individual cells. *Exp.cell research.*175, 184-191.

Ursini CL, Cavallo D, Fresegna AM, Ciervo A, Maiello R, Buresti G, Casciardi S, Tombolini F, Bellucci S, Iavicoli S. 2012. Comparative cyto-genotoxicity assessment of functionalized and pristine multiwalled carbon nanotubes on human lung epithelial cells. *Toxicol In Vitro* 26:831–840.

Win KY, Feng SS. Effects of particle size and surface coating on the cellular uptake of polymeric nanoparticles for oral delivery of anticancer drugs. *Biomaterials.* 2005; 26:2713–22.

Zakrzewska KE, Samluk A, Wierzbicki M, *et al.* Analysis of the Cytotoxicity of Carbon-Based Nanoparticles, Diamond and Graphite, in Human Glioblastoma and Hepatoma Cell Lines. Pintus G, ed. *PLoS ONE.* 2015;10(3):e0122579. doi:10.1371/journal.pone.0122579.

Innovations in Biochemical Techniques (2020) : Page no. 8-26
ASTRAL INTERNATIONAL (P) LTD., New Delhi - 110002

Chapter 2

Cellulose: Extraction, Purification, Characterization and Applications

Erumalla Venkatanagaraju, Rajshree Roy Chowdhury, Rachiraju Hema Sindhuja, Yarram Sreelekha, Bharathi N

Department of Life Sciences, CHRIST (Deemed to be University), Hosur Road, Bengaluru-560029, Karnataka, India. Email: venkatanagarajue@gmail.com

Abstract

Cellulose is proven to be a versatile biomaterial and can be employed for commercial purposes in various industries. In this paper, various extraction methods of cellulose from plants and microbial sources has been described along with structure, properties, characterization and applications. X-ray diffraction, spectroscopy and microscopic techniques like SEM and TEM were used for characterization. Mechanical treatments like ultra-sonication, homogenization, cryo-crushing or chemical methods like acid-alkali treatment, chlorination or enzymatic methods can be employed for extraction. So, understanding and improving the extraction methods will better our chances of increasing the productivity.

Keywords: *Cellulose, extraction, microbial, plants, applications.*

Introduction

Cellulose, is one of the most important and abundant natural polymer present in the plant cell wall. It constitutes major portion of cotton and wood, which in turn are resources for various commercially important products like paper, cardboard, textiles and construction materials. Cellulose acetate, rayon and cellophane are some other cellulose derivatives (Keshk *et al.* 2014). The natural process of photosynthesis plays a major role in the production of most of the available cellulose in plants with the help of the complex cellulose synthase and CesA genes and proteins but some microorganisms like bacteria, algae, fungi and tunicates produce extracellular forms of cellulose. Crystalline form of cellulose can be obtained from green algae (Habibi *et al.* 2010). Cellulose synthase complex, present on the surface is involved in the synthesis of cellulose in bacteria along with other enzymes like glucokinase, phosphoglucomutase and UDP glucose phosphorylase. Bacterial cellulose is produced as a swollen gel that is dried to form thin films and 3D network of crystalline Nano and microfibrils is obtained. Primary walls of plant cell wall show cellulose assembled into microfibrils. The production of nanocellulose from different parts of plants like that of wood pulp can be done with the help of mechanical methods like homogenization and microfluidizers. The different properties of nanofibers have been discovered like the ratio of surface area to volume, and the tensile strength which has proven to be quite high (Zhang *et al.* 2011) renewability and biodegradability (Ioelovich *et al.* 2008) these features and properties of nanofibers provides great promise for wide range of applications. Cellulose can also be produced from wastes like plant straw (Zhang *et al.* 2011). Cellulose I and cellulose II are the crystalline forms of native cellulose. Cellulose I have no inter-sheet hydrogen bonding and exists in two forms *i.e.*, cellulose Iα (seen in bacteria and algae) and cellulose Iβ (seen in plants). Interconversion may be seen during microfibril formation.

Cellulose yield depends on the production method and type of microorganism when it comes to bacterial cellulose. Production of bacterial cellulose can be achieved by two culture methods, namely agitated and static. In the static type, cellulose gets piled up into a heap on the surface of the culture as a gelatinous membrane, whereas under agitation conditions, cellulose is well dispersed in the slurry in the form of stellate, granule and fibrous strand. Agitation method is preferred for industrial production and for commercial applications. One drawback of agitation is the occurrence of mutants in cultures, which are cellulose deficient. The static method is employed to investigate cellulose production (Watanabe *et al.* 1998). Acetic acid bacteria are generally involved in production of bacterial cellulose. Gluconacetobacter species, obtained from flowers, fruits, fermented foods and vinegar exhibit highest cellulose producing capacity, while other species include Pseudomonas, Sarcina, Rhizobium and Agrobacterium (Aydin *et al.* 2009). G. xylinusis the most extensively studied and used bacteria as a producer of cellulose.

Structure and Properties of Cellulose

Cellulose fibril may be considered as a cable in which long polymeric chains made up of D-glucose exist as lengthwise strands. The sugar monomers in each chain are linked by β-1,4 glycosidic bond. β-D-glucopyranose rings adopts $a^4 C_1$ ring conformation with hydroxyl group on equatorial plane and hydrogen atoms on axial plane (Habibi *et al.* 2010). Extended fibril structures are formed as all the available hydroxyl groups of glucan chains are involved in intra and inter chain hydrogen bonding. Many of these chains are aggregated to form insoluble layered sheets (Ross *et al.* 1991).

Plant cell wall is a tough, semi permeable composite tissue formed from layered deposits of cellulose which is closely associated with lignin and hemicellulose (Nuruddin *et al.* 2011). Cellulose fibrils of plant cell wall are similar to nylon strands of fiberglass. The composition of primary and secondary cell wall consists of units of glucose of the range 8000 and about 15,000 per chain respectively.

Most of the properties that are obtained from cellulose are dependent on the chain length which is nothing but the number of glucose units that make up the polymer and degree of polymerization (Jonoobi *et al.* 2015). The microfibrils found in native cellulose are detected by electron microscopy and can further be disintegrated using ultrasonic and hydrolysis (Romling *et al.* 2015). Cellulose is highly stable and can withstand heating, stretching, strong acid and alkali (Romling *et al.* 2015). Cellulose fibrils are inelastic and highly insoluble. Their molecular configuration imparts them high tensile strength similar to that of steel (Ross *et al.* 1991).

Bacterial and plant cellulose differ in their structural and mechanical properties (Valera *et al.* 2015). One of the important differences is the absence of hemicellulose, pectin and lignin in case of bacterial cellulose which in turn makes it easy to be purified (Liu *et al.* 2011). It is considered as a functional material for several industrial applications owing to its characteristic features such as high porosity, high crystallinity, high purity, biocompatibility, unique physical properties such as high sonic velocity and Young's modulus (Trovatti *et al* 2011). Unique structural features of bacterial cellulose are responsible for these properties. Culture conditions affect the microstructure of cellulose such as crystalline polymorphism, crystallinity and degree of polymerization (Watanabe *et al.* 1998). Due to these properties, bacterial cellulose finds use in food, textile industry, medicine and pharmaceutical industry (Janarthanan *et al.* 2016).

Extraction of Cellulose from Plants

In plants the most distinct feature is their cell wall, although the plant cell wall is mainly divided into two main categories as the primary cell wall and the secondary cell wall due to the differentiated cell composition but the most important component of the cell wall is the cellulose. It has β1-4 linked glucan chains, which in turn interact among each other with the help of hydrogen bonds thereby forming a crystalline microfibril (Keegstra *et al.* 2010). Apart from cellulose plant, cell wall also contains other components such as hemicellulose, pectin, and many glycoproteins as well. The hemicellulose of the plant is known to bound with the cellulose of the plant thus giving a rigid, strong structure and function the wall, for the extraction of cellulose the removal of the bonds between cellulose and hemicellulose becomes important to get a pure form of the cellulose. The composition of the cell wall varies from plant to plant; mostly it contains approximately 40 - 55% of cellulose, about 25-40% of hemicellulose and 15-35% of lignin. The presence of cellulose within these components are in crystalline nature thus making it quite difficult to obtain and extract (Penjumras *et al.* 2014).

The isolation and extraction of cellulose based products like cellulose nanofibers (CNF) has been of great importance in the last few decades due to high demands for renewable resources, environmental issues and cause of their highly positive properties such as the ratio of surface area to volume being high, their ability to sustain high stress that is tensile strength, and low coefficient of thermal expansion (Penjumras *et al.* 2014, Chen *et al.* 2011). Although there are quite some source from cellulose the main source for CNs are the plants from their cell wall as they are more renewable and the cost of extraction is low when compared to other sources, the extraction of cellulose from plant source has been exploited by many researchers and is still going on (Chen *et al.* 2011). To avoid economic problems such as the use to food resources researches have also started using waste parts of plant or agriculture waste as a source (Nuruddin *et al.* 2011, Veeramachineni *et al.* 2016).

Various plants source have been used to extract and purify cellulose such as Durian rind (Penjumras *et al.* 2014), bamboo (Chen *et al.* 2011), corn stover (Costa *et al.* 2015), mulberry (Liu *et al.* 2011), *Phormium tenax* leaf (Fortunati *et al.* 2013), Sago Pulp (Veeramachineni *et al.* 2016), rice and oat husk (Oliveira *et al.* 2017), Sasalfibers (Morán *et al.* 2008), sugarcane bagasse (Saelee *et al.* 2014), milkweed stem (Reddy *et al.* 2009), banana (Zuluaga *et al.* 2007, Ibrahim *et al.* 2010), cotton (Ibrahim *et al.* 2010), kraft pulp (Nakagaito *et al.* 2004), pineapple leaf fibres (Cherian *et al.* 2010), soy hulls (Alemdar *et al.* 2008), hemp fiber (Wang *et al.* 2007). There were various methods that were tried and used on the process of extraction , the extraction can be basically employed in two types the mechanical treatment such as high pressure homogenization (Nakagaito *et al.* 2004), grinding, ultra-sonication, and the chemical treatments like the use of acid treatments, alkaline treatments, enzyme-assisted hydrolysis and the use of TEMPO mediated oxidation (Chen *et al.* 2011). There are other methods by which cellulose is extracted mainly from woods for the production of paper whose main component is cellulose; one of the most common method is the Kraft chemical process, which is a pulping method in which the wood is converted into wood pulp by breaking the bonds between the cellulose and hemicellulose (Santos *et al.* 2016). The idea of putting the mechanical a well as the chemical treatments together have been practised by many researchers for better results.

Penjumras*et al.* in his work has extracted cellulose from durian rind by delignification with acid sodium chlorite followed by mercerization (Penjumras *et al.* 2014). Use of agricultural waste for the extraction of cellulose was done by Nuruddin *et al.* where characterization of various things like rice straw, wheat straws and corn straws were done and cellulose extraction was carried out with the help of sulphuric acid hydrolysis (Nuruddin *et al.* 2011). Whereas Wenshuai Chen *et al.* in his work has used four different types of plant to extract and purify cellulose, this was done by the use of chemical as well as mechanical treatment like ultrasonic fibrillation (use of ultrasonic waves of about 20-25 kHz for about 30 mins) (Chen *et al.* 2011). Lin Liu *et al.* extracted the same from mulberry branch bark by using two-step chemical method, using acid and alkaline treatment resulting in better purification and about 92.60% increase in cellulose fibre (Liu *et al.* 2011). Scientist like Eliangela de Morais and Teixeira also used cotton fibres for cellulose by using sulphuric acid (De Morais Teixeira *et al.* 2010). Marta *et al.* used three different food by-products (wheat straw, brewer's spent grains and olive pomace) for cellulose by an optimised hydrolysis method (Martínez *et al.* 2015). Simone M.L. Rosa has tried to use a different kind of extraction method which involves no use of chlorine in the procedure for cellulose extraction from rice husk, in their paper they have imploded many steps for the isolation including alkaline treatment, delignification using acetic and nitric acid and ultrasonic treatment as well (Rosa *et al.* 2012). A different technique such as the steam exploded method as a pre-treatment and by the use of ultrasonic waves was tried by Maha *et al.* on corncob, banana plant, cotton stalk and cotton gin waste (Ibrahim *et al.* 2010).

A.N. Nakagaito *et al.* (Nakagaito *et al.* 2004) made high strength nanocomposites of cellulose with the help of high pressure of about 100 MPa on Kraft pulp. In 1982, Nuuttila *et al.* found out a method for continuous saccharification of plants for cellulose, this process of his work was further used in various ways several times (Nuuttila *et al.* 1984). Ping Lu *et al.* also worked with grape skin for cellulose extraction with an isolate of about 16.4% yield which includes a combination of different methodology together such as the use of acid-base dissolutions, and basic and acidic oxidation (Lu *et al.* 2012). Cellulose nanofibers were very first extracted and obtained by Herrick and Tubark and since it was newly invented, it was named as microfibrillated cellulose (MFC) (Jonoobi *et al.* 2015).

For nanocrystal, production of cellulose Beck-Candanedo *et al.* tried to estimate the effect of the ratio of acid and pulp and sulphuric acid hydrolysis time on the different properties of wood nanocrystal. They also were able to find shorter cellulose nanocrystals (CNS) which had lower dispersity index that can be obtained for a much longer period for hydrolysis, in addition to this they also were able to find that with the increase in the ratio of acid/pulp, the dimension of the nanocrystal decreases (Beck *et al.* 2005). Morlli*et al.* used balsa wood for CNC production, they obtained CNCs with a thickness of 7.5 ± 2.9 nm and length of 176 ± 68 nm. They concluded by saying that the obtained CNCs had suitable crystallinity with aspect ratio for the production of polymer nanocomposites (Morelli *et al.* 2012).

Table 1: Methods for Extraction of Cellulose from Various Plant Sources

Material	Extraction process	Cellulose (%)	References
Durian rind	Chlorination and mercerization	33.12 ± 0.108	(Habibi *et al.* 2010)
Wood	Chemical-ultrasonic	80.2 ± 4.2	(Zhang *et al.* 2011)
Bamboo	Chemical-ultrasonic	84.4 ± 1.8	(Zhang *et al.* 2011)
Wheat straw	Chemical-ultrasonic	84.1 ± 2.6	(Zhang *et al.* 2011)
Flax fibers	Chemical-ultrasonic	88.8 ± 1.5	(Zhang *et al.* 2011)
Corn stalks	FA/PFA/H_2O_2 process	89.6	(Ioelovich *et al.* 2008)
Rice straw	FA/PFA/H_2O_2 process	91.2	(Ioelovich *et al.* 2008)
Wheat straw	FA/PFA/H_2O_2 process	89	(Ioelovich *et al.* 2008)
Dhaincha	FA/PFA/H_2O_2 process	94.1	(Ioelovich *et al.* 2008)
Mulberry branch bark	Acid-alkaline treatment	92.60 ± 2.07	(Aydin *et al.* 2009)
Sago pulp	Acid treatment	93.6	(Watanabe *et al.* 1998)
OPEFB	Chemical treatment (pre-treatment as autoclave)	93.7	(Ibrahim *et al.* 2010)
Rice husk	Acid-alkaline treatment	93.1 ± 0.4	(Ibrahim *et al.* 2011)
Oats husk	Acid-alkaline treatment	94.1 ± 0.3	(Ibrahim *et al.* 2011)
Sugarcane bagasse	Steam explosion and xylanase	89.3	(Romling *et al.* 2015)
Hemp Untreated Acid treated Acid and alkali treated	H_2SO_4 hydrolysis	75.56 85.66 89.78	(Chen *et al.* 2011)
Corn stover	Chemical treatment (acid hydrolysis) and bleaching	45.5	(Costa *et al.* 2015)
Cotton white brown green	Sulphuric acid hydrolysis	97.7 ± 2.2 78.7 ± 0.4 80.3 ± 0.8 74.0 ± 2.0	(Veeramachineni *et al.* 2016)
Wheat straw Untreated Acid treated Acid and alkali treated	Cryocrushing, disintegration and homogenization	43.2 ± 0.15 61.8 ± 3.17 84.6 ± 4.41	(Penjumras *et al.* 2014)
Flax (bast) Untreated Acid treated Acid and alkali treated	Cryocrushing followed by homogenization	73 ± 3 84 ± 6 95 ± 1	(Nakagaito *et al.* 2004)
Bleached kraft pulp	Enzymatic pre-treatment, high shear refining	86	(Cherian *et al.* 2010)
Prickly pear fruits (skin)	Disintegration in a Waring blender followed by homogenization	27.0	(Alemdar *et al.* 2008)

Abbreviations: OPEFB (oil palm empty fruit branches)

Extraction of Cellulose from Bacteria

The isolation of cellulose from plants though feasible is a tedious process and requires several stages of purification as it consist of other non-cellulosic components along with the cellulose such as hemicellulose, lignin and pectin which has to be removed during the purification process (Kopania *et al.* 2012). Certain group of bacteria have the ability to produce cellulose as a by-product of sugar and carbohydrate metabolism. *Gluconacetobacterxylinum* (formerly known as *Acetobacter xylinum*), *Sarcina ventriculi, Agrobacterium tumefaciens* and *Rhizobium sp* are the most widely studied bacterial strains for their cellulose synthesizing property (Ross *et al.* 1991). The cellulose is produced by bacteria using a series of enzymatic reactions involving cellulose synthase as the key enzyme and is secreted extracellularly as ribbons or bands. The cellulose synthesized by microbes, though chemically similar is of more increased purity than that isolated from the plant species. Bacterial cellulose is now gaining many uses in the field of medicine, food industry, acoustics, paper industry, *etc.* (Keshk *et al.* 2014). Genetically engineering the microbes to control the degree of polarisation (dp) and the number of glucans will help in producing cellulose fibres with the desired strength and properties (Brown *et al.* 2004).

Gluconacetobacterxylinum is the most studied bacteria as a model organism for cellulose synthesis (Ross *et al.* 1991, Jonas *et al.* 1998). It is a purple sulphur obligate aerobe that uses the cellulose (synthesized extracellularly) as a protective covering, anchorage and floatation for gaining exposure to the atmosphere. They produce ribbon like microfibrils made up of cellulose 1 under normal conditions and band like the one structure made up of cellulose 2 occasionally. The type of cellulose produced by the bacteria differs with respect to the temperature also. *Acetobacter xylinum* (ATCC 23769) produces ribbon like cellulose at 28°C and band like cellulose at 4°C) (Hirai *et al.* 2002). The production of band like native cellulose is favoured by the high viscous growth medium and ribbon like cellulose production is brought about by the use of less viscous medium. Different grades of polyethylene glycol can be used to produce media with different viscosities. The bacterial colonies grown on Schramm-Hestrin agar plate were scraped out (centrifuged if grown in liquid media) and treated with 1% sodium hydroxide at 80°C for 30 minutes (Shibazaki *et al.* 1998) or 4% sodium hydroxide solution for 24 hours at 25°C and given a distilled water wash by centrifugation until neutral (Iwata *et al.* 1998).

A small amount of cellulase complex can be added to the culture broth to enhance the production. Addition of commercially available CP powder after certain pre-treatments like gel-filtration and ethanol precipitation also exhibits similar action. Bacterial cellulose pellicles can be purified by alkaline treatment and water content can be removed by solvent exchange and press drying (Ebrahimi *et al.* 2016).

Table 2: Extraction of cellulose from different bacterial strains

Source	Cellulose(g/L)	Reference
G. sacchari	2.7	(Trovatti *et al.* 2011)
Gluconobactersp	3.83	(Aydin *et al.* 2009)
G. xylinus	2.31	(Mikkelsen *et al.* 2009)
G. hansenii PJK (KCTC 10505 BP)	1.72 (with Oxygen)	(Jung *et al.* 2005)
G. hansenii PJK (KCTC 10505 BP)	2.50 (with ethanol)	(Park, *et al.* 2003)
Gluconacetobacter sp. RKY5	5.63	(Kim *et al.* 2006)
G. xylinus strain (K3)	3.34	(Nguyen *et al.* 2008)
G. intermedius	3.5	(Tyagi *et al.* 2013)
A. xylinum BRC 5	15.30	(Hwang *et al.* 1999)
A. xylinum BPR2001	12.00 (with fructose and agar)	(Bae *et al.* 2004)
Acetobacter sp. V6	4.16	(Son *et al.* 2003)
Acetobacter sp. A9	15.20	(Son *et al.* 2001)
A. xylinum E25	3.50	(Chao *et al.* 2001)
*A.xylinum*NUST4.1	6.00	(Zhou *et al.* 2007)
*G. xylinus*IFO 13773	10.10	(Keshk *et al.* 2006)
A.xylinum sp. sucrofermentans BPR2001	8.70 (fructose agar oxygen)	(Chao *et al.* 2000)
Co-culture of *Gluconacetobacter sp.* st-60–12 and *Lactobacillus mali* JCM1116	4.20	(Seto *et al.* 2006)

Abrevation: *A.xylinum: Acetobacter xylinum; G.sacchri: Gluconacetobactersacchari; G. hanseniiPJK (KCTC 10505 BP): Gluconacetobacter.hanseniiPJK (KCTC 10505 BP); G.xylinus strain (K3):Gluconacetobacter.xylinus strain (K3); G.intermedius; Gluconoacetobacter intermedius;A. xylinum E25:Acetobacter xylinum E25; A. xylinum BRC 5: Acetobacter xylinumBRC 5; A. xylinum BPR2001:Acetobacter xylinumBPR2001; A.xylinumNUST4.1: Acetobacter xylinumNUST4.1; G.xylinusIFO 13773:GluconacetobacterxylinusIFO 13773.*

Characterization

Characterization is one of the most important steps after extraction of cellulose from the sample. The surface morphology and microstructure of cellulosic fibres and CNCs is studied by scanning electron microscopy (SEM) while long, slender microfibrils or nanoparticles examined by transmission electron microscopy (TEM) confirms the extraction of cellulose from a particular sample to be successful. The changes caused by various treatments on the structure of sample can be established by FTIR (Fourier transform infrared microscopy) and determination of various chemical constituents of cellulose fibres can be achieved by analysis of its different forms. Images in FE-SEM (field emission scanning electron microscope) are obtained by raster scan of sample surface using high energy beam of electron. A field emission scanning electron microscope (FE-SEM) The main difference between SEM and FE-SEM is emitter type. Atomic Force Microscopy (AFM), relatively new variant of microscopy involves the use of a sharp tip for scanning the sample surface and detection is based on force of interaction between the sample and the tip. The topography and morphology of the cellulose nanocrystals are imaged using an AFM. In aqueous solutions, direct observation at high resolution can be achieved. Solids and fluids can be structurally characterized in nm range using x-ray diffraction. Intensity of diffraction of crystalline and amorphous regions was referred for calculating crystallinity index (CrI) of samples.

The characterization of cellulose from six different plants is as follows:

Rice husk composition was determined and, after each stage, the material obtained was characterized carefully. Nurain *et al.* performed various morphological investigations using TEM and SEM. Continuous elimination of non-cellulosic components was identified by FTIR. Increase in crystallinity with successive treatments was revealed by x-ray diffraction studies (Johar *et al.* 2012). Sun *et al.* studied isolated cellulose samples in sugarcane bagasse by two techniques (degradation and non-degradation) to estimate comparative crystallinity. Degradation methods included thermal analysis and acid hydrolysis whereas non-degradation methods included NMR spectroscopy, FT-IR *etc.* (Sun *et al.* 2004). Wenshuai *et al.* used ultrasonic processor to obtain cellulosic suspensions from four different plants and observed the cellulose fibres using a type of SEM called FE-SEM (Field emission SEM). Removal of lignin and hemicellulose in large amounts during chemical treatments was indicated by FTIR whereas degree of crystallinity of cellulose in cellulose nanofibers and chemically purified cellulose fibres was shown by x-ray diffraction data (Zhang *et al.* 2011).

Wilson *et al.* characterized the nanocrystals by thermal stability, crystallinity index, surface charge and morphology from soy hulls using SEM and TEM. To obtain spectra, infrared spectrophotometer (Shimadzu IR Prestige-21) was used and for total sulphur content determination, elemental analysis can be carried out followed by X-ray diffraction (Flauzino *et al.* 2013). Ping *et al.* purified cellulose from rice straw and for analysis of samples, FTIR spectroscopy was employed. The topological and microstructural details were studied by FE-SEM. He conducted sulfur mapping using the Energy-dispersive X-ray spectroscopy (EDS) and used a TEM to image CNCs. The overall crystalline phases of samples was analysed by Wide-angle X-ray diffraction (XRD). 3D simulation, image processing and section analysiswere carried out by Atomic force microscopy (AFM) (Lu *et al.* 2012). After treatment, chemical modifications in banana were characterized by using FTIR spectroscopy by Robin *et al.* Homogenization gives individual or bundled microfibrils (PH) but treatment with organosolv (PO) produces smaller aggregates (micro crystallites) of cellulose. The PO-treated sample showed sharper rings in the X-ray diffraction which suggested higher crystallinity due to dissolution of amorphous zones by the acid treatment and more efficient removal of hemicelluloses (Zuluaga *et al.* 2007).

Application of Cellulose in Various Fields

1) Drug Delivery

Since the early 1970s, the importance of drug delivery systems has reached another level in medicine especially with the use of polymers, and cellulose derivatives (Arca *et al.* 2018). Physiological barriers, drug instability, immunogenicity and delivery route often limit the drug efficiency. Consequently, enormous efforts are being made to develop drug delivery systems. On industrial scale, various techniques are being employed for production of encapsulated drugs (Zhang *et al.* 2015). Natural polymers are the most popular biomaterials used for controlled-release dosage forms and hydrophilic polymer matrix is used for extended-release dosage forms (Kamel *et al.* 2008). For production of delivery systems that are time-regulated, microcrystalline cellulose, hydroxypropyl methyl cellulose, hydroxyethyl cellulose and hydroxypropyl cellulose are used. Because of their unique biological properties, easy availability and biocompatibility, polysaccharides such as chitosan, cellulose derivatives and alginate, are the most common encapsulation agents (Zhang *et al.* 2015).

Cellulose and its derivatives especially cellulose ethers are widely used as bio adhesives and mucoadhesive. These are drugs which contain polymeric films and have ability to combine with moisture or mucous, thereby attaching themselves to biological membrane. These drugs have higher patient compliance and the ability to increase the residence time at drug absorption site. Non-ionic ether forms of cellulose like ethyl cellulose, hydroxyethyl cellulose, methylcellulose, hydroxypropyl cellulose, or hydroxypropyl methyl cellulose, carboxymethyl cellulose, and sodium carboxymethyl cellulose, an anionic ether form have been recently used in bio adhesives. These are less dependent on adhesion time and adhesion force but various other polymers can be used with ether cellulose to further reduce the dependency (Shokri *et al.* 2019). Bacterial cellulose can be used as a drug delivery material. The matrix is encapsulated with various antibiotics to act against the infection. Release of local anaesthetic, lidocaine was carried out using cellulose membranes of bacteria and it was observed that the permeation rate of the drug with the membrane was significantly lower than that of gel and aqueous solution delivery systems. Paracetamol delivery is made possible because of the ability of bacterial cellulose in forming foldable, soft and flexible films without the help of any plasticizer (DeOliveira *et al.* 2016). This suggests that the cellulose from bacterial sources can be considered as a useful material for the delivery of drugs that prolongs the release time of the drugs. Gericke *et al* suggested microencapsulation using cellulose sulphate due to its uniform sulphate group distribution, high viscosity and good water solubility (Penjumras *et al.* 2014). Wang *et al* confirmed the use of chitosan cellulose sulphate for microbial triggered drug delivery that is specific to colony (Zhang *et al.* 2015). Muller *et al.* mixed poly (ethyleneimine) with cellulose sulfate and used the compound for drug delivery (Muller *et al.* 2012).

2) Use As Nanoparticles

Nanocrystals and nanofibrils are the two classes of nanoparticles obtained from cellulose (Moon *et al.* 2013). Cellulose has high-end applications involved in water purification. Chang *et al* suggested that the nano-sized cellulose has attractive surface area, superior adsorption properties, ease of fictionalization, absence of internal diffusion and chemical accessibility (Olivera *et al.* 2016). These properties aid in adsorption of heavy m*et al*s and dyes for the water systems. Nano cellulose can be used as alternative to plastics and can reduce the use of oil and therefore ultimately acts a renewable, biodegradable material with good mechanical properties (Kontturi *et al.* 2015). Nano cellulose has high strength, low density and very high aspect ratio (nanofibrils). It is used to manufacture chiral templates, security papers, glass separators, magnetic responsive materials and sensors. Cellulose nanocrystals (CNC's) on their surface exhibit hydroxyl groups which allows surface modification, such as esterification, etherification, oxidation, silylation *etc.* These facilitate the incorporation and dispersion of nanocrystals into various polymer matrices and are therefore considered to be ideal polymer matrix nano reinforcements (Zhou *et al.* 2015). Surface Modification of cellulose nanocrystals with polymers, nanoparticles and small molecules allows them to be used as drug delivery agents in their zero-dimensional form, and contributes properties like strength, flexibility and compressibility in 1D, 2D and 3D forms respectively (Grishkewich *et al.* 2017). Modified cellulose nanocrystals are widely used as antiviral and antibacterial agents, drug-delivery vehicles, biosensors, biocatalysts, gene vectors and in various fields of tissue engineering, organic electronics and biomedical engineering. Strong dipole moment and piezoelectric properties are characteristics of CNC's obtained from wood. When these are coated with conductive polymers with poor processability and mechanical properties, composites having high strength, moderate conductivity and lower thermal expansion coefficient are produced (Grishkewich *et al.* 2017). They can be used as free radical scavengers, rheological modifiers, stabilizers for pickering emulsion, and for strengthening films for food packaging. Development of useful products by transforming cellulose nanoparticles will be a huge step in resource utilization and it also helps in reduction of carbon footprint as they are potential carbon storage units.

3) Other Medical Applications

Bacterial cellulose is considered as a highly biocompatible material. When a material is said to be biocompatible, it means that it is non-toxic to the biological system and obtains a satisfactory host response upon specific application. The complex interactions between the implant and the tissue present in close proximity determines the biocompatibility. Bacterial cellulose is structurally similar to extracellular matrix compounds such as collagen. It is non-immunogenic because of the polysaccharide nature of the cellulose (DeOliveira *et al.* 2016). It is also used to replace the burned skin and thus is extensively used in biomedical field for wound dressing. In addition to it, cellulose is non-bactericidal in nature and hence prevents infections when used for wound dressing. To improve its antimicrobial activities, cellulose has been linked with other types of antibacterial agents (DeOliveira *et al.* 2016). Sutures are the most widely used group of devices implanted into humans. Carbon based sutures have been produced by the modification of cellulose filaments (Hoenich *et al.* 2006). Ether and ester derivatives of cellulose is used to coat various pharmaceutical productssuch as tablets, microcapsules, pellets, granules and pills to protect them from oxygen, moisture, adverse environmental conditions, acidic and enzymatic degradation *etc.* (Shokri *et al.* 2019). Tablets are also coated with sodium carboxymethyl cellulose, microcrystalline cellulose, hydroxypropyl methyl cellulose, hydroxyethyl cellulose and hydroxypropyl cellulose. Hydroxypropyl cellulose and hydroxypropyl methyl cellulose in the hydrated form is used to target the drug delivery to colon after oral drug administration. These compounds swell when hydrated by gastric media and delay absorption. Hence, they are used as binders in oral drug formulations (Kamel *et al.* 2008). Methyl cellulose is used in the treatment of constipation, diverticulosis whereas ethyl cellulose has the ability to sustain release of drugs. Oxycellulose used in various surgical procedures, by direct application to the oozing surface. It is also used in the formulation of sunscreen sprays, anti-fungal cream, anti-acne cream and lotion (Lavanya *et al.* 2011).

4) Other Applications

Cellulose is used for the production of bioethanol and biohydrogen. Bioethanol reduces carbon monoxide, nitrous oxides and hydrocarbons emissions and has a higher-octane rating, vapour pressure and heat of vaporization than petroleum fuels to help engines run at higher compression ratios giving higher net performance and increased power outputs. Hydrogen production using forest biomass is a good solution for solving the energy problem. Biohydrogen can be used to upgrade bitumen for the production of synthetic crude oil (SCO) (Bogati *et al.* 2011). Cellulose rich material are feasible appropriate hydrogel precursor materials, due to their large availability, low cost and their biocompatibility. The responsiveness of some cellulosics to variations in the external stimuli where biodegradability of hydrogel is required makes it more appealing (Sannino *et al.* 2009). Methylcellulose is used for manufacturing papers and textiles. The fibers are protected from absorbing water or oil by the presence of cellulose. Pure cellulose can also be used as thickening and stabilizing agent in processed foods. The microbial cellulose due to gel-like properties and complete indigestibility in the human intestinal tract have made it an attractive food base (Chawla *et al.* 2009). Oxycellulose and sodium carboxy methylcellulose is used in numerous cosmetic, pharmaceutical, agricultural, and consumer products. Microcrystalline cellulose is used as an emulsifier, stabilizer, dispersing and anticaking agent. Carboxymethyl cellulose (CMC) in its insoluble micro granular form is used in ion-exchange chromatography as column packing material for purification and separation of proteins. It can also be used in ice packs to form a eutectic mixture resulting in a much lower freezing point with more cooling capacity than ice (Lavanya *et al.* 2011). Cellulose acetate is being used in many different textile applications due to its good textile processing performance and other useful attributes. It is used to weave fabrics, knits, braids and is often used in combination with other fibres to make yarns (Law *et al.* 2004).

Conclusion

Materials of biological origin are generally preferred over artificial products. With the help of new age technology, natural polymers can be modified and tailored to meet our needs. Cellulose finds its applications in literally every sector of our economy like drug delivery, textiles, adhesives, lubricants and biomedical industries *etc.* Though it is primarily obtained from plants, it can also be obtained from various microbes especially bacteria with added advantage of unique properties. Methods can be devised to extract cellulose from used media and other biological wastes. Extensive studies must be carried out to find out more about the biological pathways to devise various efficient means of cellulose extraction that are scalable and can be commercialized. Mutation of bacterial strains and Recombinant DNA technology can be employed for genetic manipulation leading to higher yields.

References

Alemdar, A., Sain, M., (2008). Isolation and characterization of nanofibers from agricultural residues–Wheat straw and soy hulls. *Bioresource Technology*, 99: 1664–1671.

Arca, H. C., Mosquera Giraldo, L. I., Bi, V., Xu, D., Taylor, L. S., & Edgar, K. J. (2018). Pharmaceutical Applications of Cellulose Ethers and Cellulose Ether Esters. *Biomacromolecules*, 19(7): 2351–2376. https://doi.org/10.1021/acs.biomac.8b00517

Aydin, Ya, N. D. A. (2009). Isolation of Cellulose Producing Bacteria from Wastes of Vinegar Fermentation. *Proceedings of the World Congress on Engineering and Computer Sceience*, I:20–23. https://doi.org/10.1007/s10570-010-9405-y

Bae, S., Sugano, Y., Shoda, M., (2004). Improvement of bacterial cellulose production by addition of agar in a jar fermentor. *Journal of bioscience and bioengineering* ,97: 33–38.

Beck-Candanedo, S., Roman, M., Gray, D.G., (2005). Effect of reaction conditions on the properties and behavior of wood cellulose nanocrystal suspensions. *Biomacromolecules*, 6 1048–1054.

Bhatnagar, A., Sain, M., (2005). Processing of cellulose nanofiber-reinforced composites. *Journal of Reinforced Plastics and Composites* ,24: 1259–1268.

Bogati, D. R. (2011). Cellulose Based Biochemicals and Their Applications. Saimaa University of Applied Sciences, 2–37.

Brown Jr, R.M., 2004. Cellulose structure and biosynthesis: what is in store for the 21st century? Journal of Polymer Science Part A: Polymer Chemistry, 42: 487–495.

Chao, Y., Ishida, T., Sugano, Y., Shoda, M., (2000). Bacterial cellulose production by Acetobacter xylinum in a 50-L internal-loop airlift reactor. *Biotechnology and bioengineering*, 68: 345–352.

Chao, Y., Sugano, Y., Shoda, M., (2001). Bacterial cellulose production under oxygen-enriched air at different fructose concentrations in a 50-liter, internal-loop airlift reactor. *Applied microbiology and biotechnology*, 55: 673–679.

Chawla, P. R., Bajaj, I. B., Survase, S. A., & Singhal, R. S. (2009). Microbial cellulose: Fermentative production and applications. *Food Technology and Biotechnology*, 47(2): 107–124. https://doi.org/10.1117/12.536212

Chen, W., Yu, H., Liu, Y., Hai, Y., Zhang, M., Chen, P., (2011). Isolation and characterization of cellulose nanofibers from four plant cellulose fibers using a chemical-ultrasonic process. Cellulose ,18: 433–442. https://doi.org/10.1007/s10570-011-9497-z

Cherian, B.M., Leão, A.L., de Souza, S.F., Thomas, S., Pothan, L.A., Kottaisamy, M., (2010). Isolation of nanocellulose from pineapple leaf fibres by steam explosion. *Carbohydrate Polymers*, 81: 720–725.

Costa, L., Fonseca, A.F., Pereira, F.V., Druzian, J.I., (2015). Extraction and characterization of cellulose nanocrystals from corn stover. *Cell Chem Technol* ,49: 127–133.

De Morais Teixeira, E., Corrêa, A.C., Manzoli, A., de Lima Leite, F., de Oliveira, C.R., Mattoso, L.H.C., (2010) Cellulose nanofibers from white and naturally colored cotton fibers. *Cellulose* ,17: 595–606. https://doi.org/10.1007/s10570-010-9403-0

De Oliveira Barud, H. G., da Silva, R. R., da Silva Barud, H., Tercjak, A., Gutierrez, J., Lustri, W. R., ... Ribeiro, S. J. L. (2016). A multipurpose natural and renewable polymer in medical applications: Bacterial cellulose. *Carbohydrate Polymers, 153*: 406–420. https://doi.org/10.1016/j.carbpol.2016.07.059

Ebrahimi, E., Babaeipour, V., Khanchezar, S., (2016). Effect of down-stream processing parameters on the mechanical properties of bacterial cellulose. *Iranian Polymer Journal* ,25: 739-746.

Flauzino Neto, W. P., Silvério, H. A., Dantas, N. O., & Pasquini, D. (2013). Extraction and characterization of cellulose nanocrystals from agro-industrial residue - Soy hulls. Industrial Crops and Products, 42(1): 480–488. https://doi.org/10.1016/j.indcrop.2012.06.041

Fortunati, E., Puglia, D., Monti, M., Peponi, L., Santulli, C., Kenny, J.M., Torre, L., (2013). Extraction of Cellulose Nanocrystals from Phormium tenax Fibres. *Journal of Polymers and the Environment*, 21: 319–328. https://doi.org/10.1007/s10924-012-0543-1

Grishkewich, N., Mohammed, N., Tang, J., & Tam, K. C. (2017). Recent advances in the application of cellulose nanocrystals. *Current Opinion in Colloid and Interface Science*, 29: 32–45. https://doi.org/10.1016/j.cocis.2017.01.005

Habibi, Y., Lucia, L. A., & Rojas, O. J. (2010). Cellulose Nanocrystals : Chemistry , Self-Assembly , and Applications. *Chemical Reviews*, 110: 3479–3500.

Habibi, Y., Mahrouz, M., Vignon, M.R., (2009). Microfibrillated cellulose from the peel of prickly pear fruits. *Food Chemistry* ,115: 423–429.

Hirai, A., Tsuji, M., Horii, F., (2002). TEM study of band-like cellulose assemblies produced by Acetobacter xylinum at 4 C. Cellulose ,9: 105–113.

Hoenich, N. (2006). Cellulose for Medical Applications Past, Present, And Future. *BioResources,* 1: 270–280.

Hwang, J.W., Yang, Y.K., Hwang, J.K., Pyun, Y.R., Kim, Y.S., (1999). Effects of pH and dissolved oxygen on cellulose production by Acetobacter xylinum BRC5 in agitated culture. *Journal of Bioscience and Bioengineering* , 88: 183–188.

Ibrahim, m.m., agblevor, f.a., el-zawawy, w.k., (2010). Isolation and characterization of cellulose and lignin from steam-exploded lignocellulosic biomass ,22

Ioelovich. (2008). Nanostructured cellulose: Review. *BioResources* 3(4): 1403-1418

Iwata, T., Indrarti, L., Azuma, J.-I., (1998). Affinity of hemicellulose for cellulose produced by Acetobacter xylinum. *Cellulose,* 5: 215–228.

Janardhnan, S., Sain, M.M., (2007). Isolation of cellulose microfibrils–an enzymatic approach. *Bioresources,* 1: 176–188.

Janarthanan, P., Veeramachineni, A., Langford, S., Muniyandy, S., Sathasivam, T., & Yan, L. (2016). Optimizing Extraction of Cellulose and Synthesizing Pharmaceutical Grade Carboxymethyl Sago Cellulose from Malaysian Sago Pulp. *Applied Sciences,* 6(6): 170. https://doi.org/10.3390/app6060170

Johar, N., Ahmad, I., & Dufresne, A. (2012). Extraction, preparation and characterization of cellulose fibres and nanocrystals from rice husk. *Industrial Crops and Products,* 37(1): 93–99. https://doi.org/10.1016/j.indcrop.2011.12.016

Jonas, R., Farah, L.F., (1998). Production and application of microbial cellulose. *Polymer Degradation and Stability,* 59: 101–106.

Jonoobi, M., Oladi, R., Davoudpour, Y., Oksman, K., Dufresne, A., Hamzeh, Y., & Davoodi, R. (2015). Different preparation methods and properties of nanostructured cellulose from various natural resources and residues: a review. *Cellulose,* 22(2): 935–969. https://doi.org/10.1007/s10570-015-0551-0

Jonoobi, M., Oladi, R., Davoudpour, Y., Oksman, K., Dufresne, A., Hamzeh, Y., Davoodi, R., (2015). Different preparation methods and properties of nanostructured cellulose from various natural resources and residues: a review. *Cellulose,* 22: 935–969. https://doi.org/10.1007/s10570-015-0551-0

Jung, J.Y., Park, J.K., Chang, H.N., (2005). Bacterial cellulose production by Gluconacetobacter hansenii in an agitated culture without living non-cellulose producing cells. *Enzyme and Microbial Technology,* 37: 347–354.

Kamel, S., Ali, N., Jahangir, K., Shah, S. M., & El-Gendy, A. A. (2008). Pharmaceutical significance of cellulose: A review. *Express Polymer Letters,* 2(11): 758–778. https://doi.org/10.3144/expresspolymlett.2008.90

Keegstra, K., (2010). Plant Cell Walls. PLANT PHYSIOLOGY, 154: 483–486. https://doi.org/10.1104/pp.110.161240

Keshk, S. M. (2014). Bacterial Cellulose Production and its Industrial Applications. *Journal of Bioprocessing & Biotechniques,* 04(02). https://doi.org/10.4172/2155-9821.1000150

Keshk, S., Sameshima, K., (2006). Influence of lignosulfonate on crystal structure and productivity of bacterial cellulose in a static culture. *Enzyme and Microbial Technology* , 40: 4–8.

Kim, S.-Y., Kim, J.-N., Wee, Y.-J., Park, D.-H., Ryu, H.-W., (2006). Production of bacterial cellulose by *Gluconacetobacter* sp. RKY5 isolated from persimmon vinegar. *Presented at the Twenty-seventh symposium on biotechnology for fuels and chemicals*, Springer, pp. 705–715.

Kopania, E., Wietecha, ., Ciechańska, D., (2012). Studies on isolation of cellulose fibres from waste plant biomass. *Fibres & Textiles in Eastern Europe.*

Lavanya, D., Kulkarni, P. K., Dixit, M., Raavi, P. K., & Krishna, L. N. V. (2011). Sources of Cellulose and Their Applications – a Review. *International Journal of Drug Formulation and Research*, 2(6): 19–38.

Law, R. C. (2004). 5. Applications of cellulose acetate— 5.1 Cellulose acetate in textile application. *Macromolecular Symposia*, 208(1): 255–266. https://doi.org/10.1002/masy.200450410

Liu, L., Jiang, T., & Yao, J. (2011). A Two-Step Chemical Process for the Extraction of Cellulose Fiber and Pectin from Mulberry Branch Bark Efficiently. *Journal of Polymers and the Environment*, 19(3): 568–573. https://doi.org/10.1007/s10924-011-0300-x

Liu, L., Jiang, T., Yao, J., (2011). A Two-Step Chemical Process for the Extraction of Cellulose Fiber and Pectin from Mulberry Branch Bark Efficiently. *Journal of Polymers and the Environment*, 19: 568–573. https://doi.org/10.1007/s10924-011-0300-x

Lu, P., & Hsieh, Y. Lo. (2012). Preparation and characterization of cellulose nanocrystals from rice straw. Carbohydrate Polymers, 87(1): 564–573. https://doi.org/10.1016/j.carbpol.2011.08.022

Lu, P., Hsieh, Y.-L., (2012). Cellulose isolation and core–shell nanostructures of cellulose nanocrystals from chardonnay grape skins. *Carbohydrate Polymers*, 87: 2546–2553.

Martínez-Sanz, M., Vicente, A.A., Gontard, N., Lopez-Rubio, A., Lagaron, J.M., (2015). On the extraction of cellulose nanowhiskers from food by-products and their comparative reinforcing effect on a polyhydroxybutyrate-co-valerate polymer. *Cellulose*, 22: 535–551. https://doi.org/10.1007/s10570-014-0509-7

Mikkelsen, D., Flanagan, B.M., Dykes, G., Gidley, M., (2009). Influence of different carbon sources on bacterial cellulose production by Gluconacetobacter xylinus strain ATCC 53524. *Journal of Applied Microbiology*, 107: 576–583.

Morán, J.I., Alvarez, V.A., Cyras, V.P., Vázquez, A., (2008). Extraction of cellulose and preparation of nanocellulose from sisal fibers. *Cellulose* ,15: 149–159. https://doi.org/10.1007/s10570-007-9145-9

Morelli, C.L., Marconcini, J.M., Pereira, F.V., Bretas, R.E.S., Branciforti, M.C., (2012). Extraction and characterization of cellulose nanowhiskers from balsa wood. *Presented at the Macromolecular Symposia, Wiley Online Library,* pp. 191–195.

Muller, M., & Kebler, B. (2012). Release of pamidronate from poly(ethyleneimine)/cellulose sulphate complex nanoparticle films: An in situ ATR-FTIR study. *Journal of Pharmaceutical and Biomedical Analysis,* 66: 183–190. https://doi.org/10.1016/j.jpba.2012.03.047.

Nakagaito, A.N., Yano, H., (2004). The effect of morphological changes from pulp fiber towards nano-scale fibrillated cellulose on the mechanical properties of high-strength plant fiber based composites. *Applied Physics A: Materials Science & Processing,* 78: 547–552. https://doi.org/10.1007/s00339-003-2453-5

Nazir, M.S., Wahjoedi, B.A., Yussof, A.W., Abdullah, M.A., (2013). Eco-Friendly Extraction and Characterization of Cellulose from Oil Palm Empty Fruit Bunches. *BioResources,* 8: https://doi.org/10.15376/biores.8.2.2161-2172

Nguyen, V.T., Flanagan, B., Gidley, M.J., Dykes, G.A., (2008). Characterization of cellulose production by a *Gluconacetobacter xylinus* strain from Kombucha. *Current Microbiology,* 57: 449.

Nuruddin, M., Chowdhury, A., Haque, S. A., Rahman, M., Farhad, S. F., Jahan, M. S., & Quaiyyum, A. (2011). Extraction and chracterisation of cellulose microfibrils from agricultural wastes in integrated biorefinery initiative. *Cellulose Chemistry and Technology.,* 45(5–6): 347–354.

Nuuttila, A.I., Pohjola, V.J., (1984). Method for continuous saccharification of cellulose of plant raw material.

Oliveira, J.P. de, Bruni, G.P., Lima, K.O., Halal, S.L.M.E., Rosa, G.S. da, Dias, A.R.G., Zavareze, E. da R., (2017). Cellulose fibers extracted from rice and oat husks and their application in hydrogel. *Food Chemistry,* 221: 153–160. https://doi.org/10.1016/j.foodchem.2016.10.048

Olivera, S., Muralidhara, H. B., Venkatesh, K., Guna, V. K., Gopalakrishna, K., & Kumar K., Y. (2016). Potential applications of cellulose and chitosan nanoparticles/composites in wastewater treatment: A review. *Carbohydrate Polymers,* 153: 600–618. https://doi.org/10.1016/j.carbpol.2016.08.017

Park, J.K., Jung, J.Y., Park, Y.H., (2003). Cellulose production by Gluconacetobacter hansenii in a medium containing ethanol. *Biotechnology letters,* 25: 2055–2059.

Penjumras, P., Rahman, R.B.A., Talib, R.A., Abdan, K., (2014). Extraction and Characterization of Cellulose from Durian Rind. *Agriculture and Agricultural Science Procedia,* 2: 237–243. https://doi.org/10.1016/j.aaspro.2014.11.034

Reddy, N., Yang, Y., (2009). Extraction and characterization of natural cellulose fibers from common milkweed stems. *Polymer Engineering & Science,* 49: 2212–2217. https://doi.org/10.1002/pen.21469

Romling, U., & Galperin, M. Y. (2015). Bacterial cellulose biosynthesis: Diversity of operons, subunits, products, and functions. *Trends in Microbiology*, 23(9): 545–557. https://doi.org/10.1016/j.tim.2015.05.005

Rosa, S.M.L., Rehman, N., de Miranda, M.I.G., Nachtigall, S.M.B., Bica, C.I.D., (2012). Chlorine-free extraction of cellulose from rice husk and whisker isolation. *Carbohydrate Polymers*, 87: 1131–1138. https://doi.org/10.1016/j.carbpol.2011.08.084

Ross, P., Mayer, R., & Benziman, A. N. D. M. (1991). Cellulose Biosynthesis and Function in Bacteria. *Microbiological reviews*, 55(1): 35–58.

Saelee, K., Yingkamhaeng, N., Nimchua, T., Sukyai, P., (2014). Extraction and characterization of cellulose from sugarcane bagasse by using environmentally friendly method. Presented at the Proceedings of the 26th Annual Meeting of the Thai Society for Biotechnology and *International Conference, Mae Fah Lunag University (School of Science), Thailand*, pp. 26–29.

Sannino, A., Demitri, C., & Madaghiele, M. (2009). Biodegradable cellulose-based hydrogels: Design and applications. *Materials*, 2(2): 353–373. https://doi.org/10.3390/ma2020353

Santos, F.A. dos, Iulianelli, G.C.V., Tavares, M.I.B., (2016). The Use of Cellulose Nanofillers in Obtaining Polymer Nanocomposites: Properties, Processing, and Applications. *Materials Sciences and Applications*, 07: 257–294. https://doi.org/10.4236/msa.2016.75026

Seto, A., Saito, Y., Matsushige, M., Kobayashi, H., Sasaki, Y., Tonouchi, N., Tsuchida, T., Yoshinaga, F., Ueda, K., Beppu, T., (2006). Effective cellulose production by a coculture of *Gluconacetobacter xylinus* and *Lactobacillus mali. Applied microbiology and biotechnology*, 73: 915–921.

Shibazaki, H., Saito, M., Kuga, S., Okano, T., (1998). Native cellulose II production by Acetobacter xylinum under physical constraints. *Cellulose*, 5: 165–173.

Shokri, J., Adibki, K. (2019). Application of Cellulose and Cellulose Derivatives in Pharmaceutical Industries.

Son, H., Heo, M., Kim, Y., Lee, S., (2001). Optimization of fermentation conditions for the production of bacterial cellulose by a newly isolated Acetobacter. *Biotechnology and Applied Biochemistry*, 33: 1–5.

Son, H.-J., Kim, H.-G., Kim, K.-K., Kim, H.-S., Kim, Y.-G., Lee, S.-J., (2003). Increased production of bacterial cellulose by *Acetobacter* sp. V6 in synthetic media under shaking culture conditions. *Bioresource Technology*, 86: 215–219.

Sun, J. X., Sun, X. F., Zhao, H., & Sun, R. C. (2004). Isolation and characterization of cellulose from sugarcane bagasse. *Polymer Degradation and Stability*, 84(2): 331–339. https://doi.org/10.1016/j.polymdegradstab.2004.02.008

Trovatti, E., Serafim, L. S., Freire, C. S. R., Silvestre, A. J. D., & Neto, C. P. (2011). Gluconacetobacter sacchari: An efficient bacterial cellulose cell-factory. *Carbohydrate Polymers*, 86(3): 1417–1420. https://doi.org/10.1016/j.carbpol.2011.06.046

Tyagi, N., Suresh, S., (2013). Isolation and characterization of cellulose producing bacterial strain from orange pulp. Presented at the Advanced Materials Research, Trans Tech Publ, pp. 475–479.

Valera, M. J., Torija, M. J., Mas, A., & Mateo, E. (2015). Cellulose production and cellulose synthase gene detection in acetic acid bacteria. *Applied Microbiology and Biotechnology,* 99(3): 1349–1361. https://doi.org/10.1007/s00253-014-6198-1

Veeramachineni, A., Sathasivam, T., Muniyandy, S., Janarthanan, P., Langford, S., Yan, L., (2016). Optimizing Extraction of Cellulose and Synthesizing Pharmaceutical Grade Carboxymethyl Sago Cellulose from Malaysian Sago Pulp. *Applied Sciences,* 6: 170. https://doi.org/10.3390/app6060170

Wang, B., Sain, M., Oksman, K., (2007). Study of structural morphology of hemp fiber from the micro to the nanoscale. *Applied Composite Materials,* 14: 89.

Watanabe, K., Tabuchi, M., Morinaga, Y., & Yoshinaga, F. (1998). Structural features andproperties of bacterial cellulose produced in agitated culture. *Cellulose,* 5(3): 187–200. https://doi.org/10.1023/A:1009272904582

Zhang, M., Yu, H., Hai, Y., Chen, P., Chen, W., & Liu, Y. (2011). Isolation and characterization of cellulose nanofibers from four plant cellulose fibers using a chemical-ultrasonic process. *Cellulose,* 18(2): 433–442. https://doi.org/10.1007/s10570-011-9497-z

Zhang, Q., Lin, D., & Yao, S. (2015). Review on biomedical and bioengineering applications of cellulose sulfate. *Carbohydrate Polymers,* 132: 311–322. https://doi.org/10.1016/j.carbpol.2015.06.041

Zhou, C., Wu, Q. Recent Development in Applications of Cellulose Nanocrystals for Advanced Polymer-Based Nanocomposites by Novel Fabrication Strategies.

Zhou, L., Sun, D., Hu, L., Li, Y., Yang, J., (2007). Effect of addition of sodium alginate on bacterial cellulose production by Acetobacter xylinum. *Journal of industrial microbiology & biotechnology,* 34: 483.

Zuluaga, R., Putaux, J.-L., Restrepo, A., Mondragon, I., Gañán, P., (2007). Cellulose microfibrils from banana farming residues: isolation and characterization. *Cellulose,* 14: 585–592. https://doi.org/10.1007/s10570-007-9118-z.

Innovations in Biochemical Techniques (2020) : Page no. 27-51
ASTRAL INTERNATIONAL (P) LTD., New Delhi - 110002

Chapter 3

Bt Gene Cry1X Evaluation Against Two Targeted Insect Pests in TMV-2 Groundnut Crop

Keshamma, E

Department of Biochemistry, PG and Research Centre, Maharani's Science College for Women, Palace Road, Bangalore – 560 001.

Abstract

The transgenic plants of groundnut (*Arachis hypogeae*) cv. TMV-2 expressing a chimeric Bt gene, CrylX were generated using an *Agrobacterium tumefaciens*-mediated transformation system via *in planta* transformation strategy. A tissue culture-independent transformation method, *in planta* which targets the *Agrobacterium tumefaciens* to the apical meristem was used in the study. The purpose of this study was to prevent yield losses in groundnut crop due to the attack of major insect pests called *Helicoverpa armigera* and *Spodoptera litura*. The investigation was aimed to over express a Bt gene Cry1X in transgenic groundnut and evaluate its resistance towards targeted pests. The protocaol involves *in planta* inoculation of the embryo axes of the germinating seeds and allowing them to grow into seedlings ex vitro. PCR analysis indicated the putative transgenic nature of the T1 generation plants. Bioassays against two major pests of the groundnut, *Helicoverpa armigera* and *Spodoptera litura* revealed several T1 plants that perform well against both the larvae. This revealed that 22% of T1 plants harbour the transgene. The seeds of T1 plants when allowed to continue into the next generation amplified the gene of interest in most of the plants tested. Enzyme Linked-Immuno Sorbent Assay (ELISA) was used to identify the high expressing plants. The appearance of the protein band in the quick stick confirmed the expression of the chimeric Bt toxin. Southern analysis of 10 high expressing plants confirmed the integration of the transgene. The study also showed that the groundnut plants harbouring the Cry1X gene were resistant to two major insect defoliators of the crop and its potential would be discussed in detail. These results suggest that the chimeric Bt gene was functional in the transgenic groundnut and was being expressed.

Keywords *Arachis hypogeae, Helicoverpa armigera, Spodoptera litura,* Transgenics, in-planta, tissue culture-independent plant regeneration, synthetic cry gene.

Introduction

Groundnut/peanut (*Arachis hypogaea* L.) is an important oilseed crop of the world. Hence improvement of these crops for insect pest resistance will be an important contribution. These crops suffer from attack of large number of insect pests which are responsible for the yield loss. The major pests that attack these crops are Gram caterpillar (*Helicoverpa armigera*), Tobacco Caterpillar (*Spodoptera litura*), Red Headed Hairy Caterpillar (*Amsacta albistriga*), Leaf miner (*Aproaerema modicella*), Jassids, Thrips, Termites, Stem borers and Mites, that attack the shoot portion and the pod. This in fact is one of the important limitations for improving the productivity of pulses in general and field bean in particular (Brahmaprakash *et al.*, 2004). Hence, it is essential to develop a mechanism of pest management that does not call for explicit investment on the part of the farmer. Seed borne solutions in the form of insect resistant varieties would thus help greatly alleviate the problem. The important pests being Lepidopterans, development of insect resistant transgenics would be an important option.

Agrobacterium-mediated transformation has made a great contribution to crop improvement. Various genes that are responsible for important agronomic traits are being introduced into crop plants through the T-DNA. Plant transformation via *Agrobacterium.* Plant transformation has proven to be vital in attempts to define DNA sequence elements important for directing tissue specific and developmentally-regulated expression of promoter in addition to achieving the expression of foreign genes and determining what novel phenotype they might impose on the plant. Moreover, plants engineered to contain novel traits have been proposed to be of future agricultural benefit as this allows agronomically important traits into plants. Moreover, this technology may allow these traits to be transferred directly to breeding lines, which are currently in use, potentially reducing the time required to produce an elite line. Several traits, which may be transferred into plants using recombinant DNA technology, have been identified as having potential agronomic benefit.

A large variety of genes in the *cry* family of *Bt* delta-endotoxins such as *cry*1Ab, *cry*1Ac, *cry*2Aa, *cry*2Ab, *and Vip*3A are known to be effective against *Helicoverpa armigera* and many have already been used successfully for development of resistant transgenics (Liao *et al.*, 2002). But yet all the methods are not equally amenable for use with all the crops. For example, many crops are not easily tissue cultured and many methods of plant transformation with foreign genes depend on the development of explants from tissue culture methods. Most economically important plants are recalcitrant and not amenable to tissue culture regeneration. Therefore, there is a need to adopt for the transformation of such recalcitrant crop plants. Many crops like field bean, cotton, groundnut, safflower, sunflower, pigeon pea and capsicum are fall in this category of recalcitrant crop.

Presently, there is a considerable interest in developing plant transformation methods that excludes tissue culture steps and relies on simple protocols. These methods are called *in planta* transformation protocols.

To tackle the problems pertaining to regeneration in the above crops and certain other recalcitrant crops, alternate methods to minimize or eliminate the steps of regeneration are being standardized. These are called the *in planta* transformation protocols. Research with *Arabidopsis* has benefited from the development of high throughput transformation methods that avoid plant tissue culture (Azipiroz-Leehan and Feldmann, 1997). In particular, the development of the *Agrobacterium tumefaciens*-mediated vacuum infiltration method (Bechtold *et al.*, 1993) has had a major impact on *Arabidopsis* research. One such viable *in planta* transformation protocol has also been standardized for other cops (Rohini and Sankara Rao, 2001; 2000a; 2000b; 1999). The strategy essentially involves *in planta* inoculation of embryo axes of germination seeds and allowing them to grow into seedlings *ex vitro*. (An *Agrobacterium tumefaciens*-mediated Gene transfer method to overcome recalcitrance in Cotton (*Gossypium hirsutum*. L., "Journal of Cotton Science"- "Physiology and Molecular Biology of Plants" by Keshamma *et al*, 2008). (S. Sundaresha *et al.*, 2010). These *in planta* transformation protocols are advantageous over other methods because they do not involve regeneration procedures and therefore the tissue culture-induced somaclonal variations are avoided (Transformability in Field bean (uidA::nptII) by *Agrobacterium tumefaciens*-mediated in planta strategy. J. Plant Biol. Vol. 35 (1), April, 2008, pp 1-37 by (E. Keshamma *et al.*, 2008). (*In planta* transformation of pigeon pea : a method to overcome recalcitrance of the crop to regeneration in vitro, Phyiol. Mol. Plants, 2008: 14 (4) : 321-328 by (K. Shankar Rao *et al.*, 2008). *Agrobacterium-mediated in planta* transformation of Field bean and Recovery of stable transgenic plants expressing the cry1AcF gene, Plant Molecular Biology Reporter by (Keshamma *et al.*, 2012).

Major focus of this study was to develop efficient *in planta* transformation protocol in groundnut and subsequently to develop transgenics relevant to target insects.

Therefore, the present work envisages transforming a suitable *cry* gene and marker genes into groundnut by *Agrobacterium*-mediated *in planta* transformation. Development of these crops with enhanced insect resistance is highly warranted. Successful introduction of *cry* gene and marker genes into indigenous varieties would mark a milestone. An attempt in this direction of study would yield a new knowledge. Given this scenario, pest and disease resistant transgenic plants in the above-said crops hold tremendous promise in the management of these maladies and would serve as tremendous boon for marginal and small farmers who cannot afford to invest on pest management measures.

Very few attempts have been made towards development of *Bt* transgenics by *in planta* transformation protocol in groundnut in India. Discovery of novel *Bts* and *cry* proteins/genes will enhance our repertoire of insect protection measures in future. Based on this background, the present investigation is contemplated with the following objectives;

Objectives

1. Development of transgenic plants in groundnut for insect pest resistance using *cry*1X gene.
2. Evaluation of the transgenics.
   - Molecular analysis for the presence/integration of the *cry*1Xgene.
   - ELISA and strip tests for the expression of the *cry*1Xgene.
   - Bioassay for the efficacy of the *cry*1Xgene.

Material and Methods

Plant Material

Groundnut variety TMV-2 seeds were soaked overnight in distilled water and were surface sterilized first with 1% Bavistin for 10-15 mins and later with 0.1% $HgCl_2$ for 5-10 seconds. Then the seeds were washed thoroughly with distilled water. The seeds were later put for germination in petriplates at 28-30°C. Two-day old seedlings were taken as *ex plants* for *Agrobacterium* infection.

Bacterial Strain and vector

Agrobacterium tumefaciens strain EHA105, harbouring the binary vector, pBinBt8, was used for transformation. The vector harbours the *cry*1X and *npt*II as the genes of interest and the selectable marker, respectively **(Fig 1(a)(b) & (c))**. *Agrobacterium* strain EHA105/pBinBt8 was grown overnight at 28-30°C in LB medium (pH 7.0) containing 60 μgml^{-1} kanamycin. The bacterial culture was later resuspended in 100 ml of Winans' AB medium (pH 5.2) (Winans *et al.*, 1998) and grown for 18-20 h. For *vir* gene induction treatments, wounded tobacco leaf extract (2 g in 2 ml sterile water) was added separately to the *Agrobacterium* suspension in Winans' AB medium, 5-6 h before infection (Cheng *et al.*, 1996).

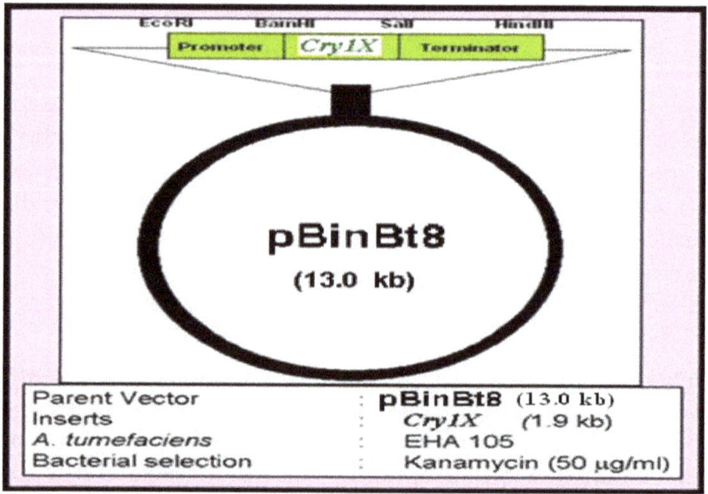

Fig 1(a): Map of the binary vector pBinBt8 (13 kb).

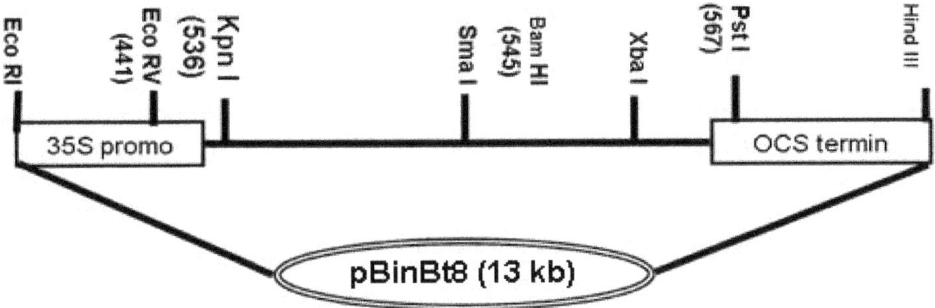

Fig 1(b): The genomic map of the plasmid pBinBt8 (13 kb) showing the inserts and the restriction fragments of the inserts amenable for digestion.

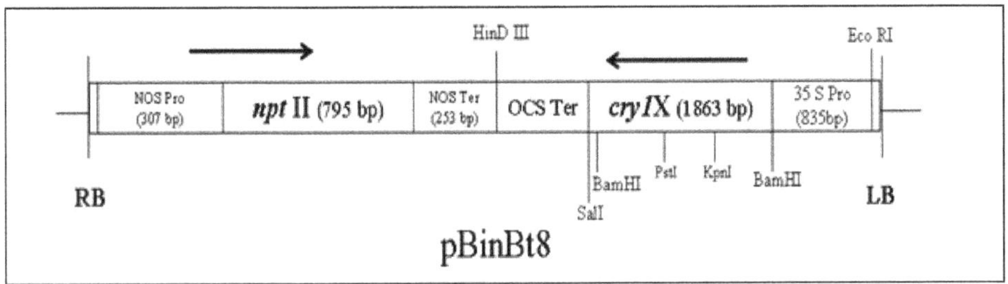

Fig 1(c): T-DNA map of the binary vector pBinBt8 (13 kb) carrying *cry*1X and *npt*II genes.

Transformation and Recovery of Transformants

Groundnut cv.TMV-2 variety transformation and generation of the primary transformants was accomplished using the tissue-culture independent *in planta* transformation procedure. The seedlings with just emerging plumule were infected by pricking at the meristem with a sterile needle and subsequent immersion in the culture of *Agrobacterium* for 16-22 h. Following infection, the seedlings were washed briefly with sterile water and the seedlings were later transferred to autoclaved soilrite (vermiculite equivalent) moistened with water for germination under aseptic conditions in the growth room in wide mouth capped glass jars of 250 ml capacity, 5 seedlings per jar. After 5 to 6 days, the seedlings were transferred to soilrite in pots and were allowed to grow under growth room conditions for at least 12 days before they were transferred to the greenhouse. The growth chamber was maintained at 28°C under a 14 h photoperiod with florescent light of intensity 35 μmol m^{-2} s^{-1}.

Molecular Analyses of the Putative Transgenic Plants

Tissues from the progeny plants were analyzed for the presence of the introduced genes. Genomic DNA was isolated following the procedure of Dellaporta *et al.* (1983) from fresh leaf tissue of the greenhouse-grown T_1 generation plants that was used for PCR, grid PCR with individual plant samples and Southern blot.

Grid PCR Analyses of Putative Transgenic Plants in T_1 Generation

Seeds from each individual plant were maintained as separate lines. T_1 groundnut plants were grown in greenhouse following recommended package of practices (Anonymous, 2000). Plants were labeled with aluminium tags. They were divided into different grids containing 100 plants each such that 10 plants each along the rows or columns could be counted. Samples from each such 10 plants either along the row or along the column formed a composite sample. As a result, from each grid of 100 plants numbered from 1 to 100, 20 composite samples originated.

Genomic DNA from composite samples was isolated by CTAB method as mentioned earlier. PCR analysis of composite samples was done using specific primers under standardized PCR conditions. PCR was also performed to confirm the presence of the gene in the plants that were selected to be advanced further. PCR was performed to amplify 750 bp *npt*II gene fragment in the putative transformants. In order to amplify the *npt*II gene fragment, PCR was initiated by a hot start at 94°C for 4 min followed by 32 cycles of 1 min at 94°C, 1 min 30 s at 58°C and 1 min at 72°C. PCR was also performed with the gene specific primers (*cry*1Xgene) to amplify a 950 bp fragment. The conditions for the reaction were same as above. The product was run on a 1% agarose gel.

Southern Analysis

In order to analyse the total genomic DNA for transgene integration of *cry*1X gene, 15 μg of total genomic DNA was digested with the appropriate restriction enzyme. Both the digested and uncut DNA samples were electrophoresed on a 0.8% agarose gel. The separated fragments along with the uncut DNA were transferred onto a nylon membrane and hybridized with a labeled 950 bp PCR amplified product of the *cry*1Xgene. Hybridization was performed at 65°C in Church buffer for 18 h. Membranes were washed for 30 min each in 2X SSC, 0.1% SDS; 0.1X SSC, 0.1% SDS at 65°C (Sambrook *et al.*, 1989). The blots were exposed to a phosphoimager.

Expression Analyses of the Putative Transgenic Plants

Enzyme Linked Immuno Sorbent Assay (ELISA)

Qualitative ELISA was used to check the *cry* protein produced in the transgenic groundnut plants. A *cry*1AB/*cry*1Ac plate kit (Envirologix Inc, Portland, USA) was used for this purpose. The Sandwich ELISA was performed according to the manufacturer's instructions.

Quick Dip Stick Detection

Quick detection of the hybrid/fused *Bt* protein was done using the "*cry*1Ab/*cry*1Ac lateral flow Quickstix Strip" as per the manufacturer's instructions (*Bt* Quant, Nagpur, India). The presence of a test line (second line) on the membrane strip between the control line (common to all, including the non-transformed control) and the protective tape would indicate the expression of foreign *Bt* protein in the transgenics.

In vitro Insect Bioassay

All bioassays were performed on detached, fully expanded, groundnut leaves. Two trifoliate leaves were collected from each selected plant and washed with distilled water. The leaves were wiped clean of all dirt and other debris. The stalks of the leaves were wrapped with wet cotton pieces and placed in a plastic container. Ten neonate larvae of *H. armigera/S. litura* were released on to each leaf. Observations were recorded daily for a period of four days on the number of dead and live larvae, per cent of leaf damage and the leaf condition. The containers were wiped clean daily.

Statistical Analyses

Data were analysed using MS excel and SPSS software. Means and standard deviations were worked out for all values depending on the need. The mean values of all the plant parameters were subjected to ANOVA (Sokal and Rohlf 1969). Correlation and regression analyses were done following by (Snedecor and Cochram (1967). Scatter plots, frequency distribution graphs were generated where necessary for representing the data.

Results

In Planta Transformation of Groundnut Variety tmv-2 With *cry*1x Gene

Approximately 50 seedlings were subjected to *in planta* transformation. Twenty five of these plants survived after shifting to the pots in the greenhouse. Under the greenhouse conditions, the plants grew normally, flowered and set pods. These plants were designated as the T_0 generation plants. Seeds were harvested and used for raising the T_1 generation plants.

Analysis of the T_1 Generation Plants

As many as 650 seeds were harvested from 25 primary transformants out of which 450 T_1 plants could be established in the greenhouse. Among these, 400 healthy plants were selected for analysis and were divided into groups of 100 as grids to form 80 composite samples for PCR analysis (Fig 2).

Composite samples	11 ↓	12 ↓	13 ↓	14 ↓	15 ↓	16 ↓	17 ↓	18 ↓	19 ↓	20 ↓
1 →	1	2	3	4	5	6	7	8	9	10
2 →	11	12	13	14	15	16	17	18	19	20
3 →	21	22	23	24	25	26	27	28	29	30
4 →	31	32	33	34	35	36	37	38	39	40
5 →	41	42	43	44	45	46	47	48	49	50
6 →	51	52	53	54	55	56	57	58	59	60
7 →	61	62	63	64	65	66	67	68	69	70
8 →	71	72	73	74	75	76	77	78	79	80
9 →	81	82	83	84	85	86	87	88	89	90
10→	91	92	93	94	95	96	97	98	99	100

Composite samples	31 ↓	32 ↓	33 ↓	34 ↓	35 ↓	36 ↓	37 ↓	38 ↓	39 ↓	40 ↓
21→	101	102	103	104	105	106	107	108	109	110
22→	111	112	113	114	115	116	117	118	119	120
23→	121	122	123	124	125	126	127	128	129	130
24→	131	132	133	134	135	136	137	138	139	140
25→	141	142	143	144	145	146	147	148	149	150
26→	151	152	153	154	155	156	157	158	159	160
27→	161	162	163	164	165	166	167	168	169	170
28→	171	172	173	174	175	176	177	178	179	180
29→	181	182	183	184	185	186	187	188	189	190
30→	191	192	193	194	195	196	197	198	199	200

Composite samples	51 ↓	52 ↓	53 ↓	54 ↓	55 ↓	56 ↓	57 ↓	58 ↓	59 ↓	60 ↓
41→	201	202	203	204	205	206	207	208	209	210
42→	211	212	213	214	215	216	217	218	219	220
43→	221	222	223	224	225	226	227	228	229	230
44→	231	232	233	234	235	236	237	238	239	240
45→	241	242	243	244	245	246	247	248	249	250
46→	251	252	253	254	255	256	257	258	259	260
47→	261	262	263	264	265	266	267	268	269	270
48→	271	272	273	274	275	276	277	278	279	280
49→	281	282	283	284	285	286	287	288	289	290
50→	291	292	293	294	295	296	297	298	299	300

Composite samples	71 ↓	72 ↓	73 ↓	74 ↓	75 ↓	76 ↓	77 ↓	78 ↓	79 ↓	80 ↓
61→	301	302	303	304	305	306	307	308	309	310
52→	311	312	313	314	315	316	317	318	319	320
63→	321	322	323	324	325	326	327	328	329	330
64→	331	332	333	334	335	336	337	338	339	340
65→	341	342	343	344	345	346	347	348	349	350
66→	351	352	353	354	355	356	357	358	359	360
67→	361	362	363	364	365	366	367	368	369	370
68→	371	372	373	374	375	376	377	378	379	380
69→	381	382	383	384	385	386	387	388	389	390
70→	391	392	393	394	395	396	397	398	399	400

Numbers in — Composits samples
Number in red— Putative transgenics
Numbers in black — Escapes/ Non Transformed plants

Fig 2: Grid PCR alignment of putative T_1*cry*1X transgenic groundnut plants using *npt*II primers.

Molecular Analysis by Grid PCR

PCR analysis with *npt*II specific primers of the 80 grid samples revealed the possibility of presence of the gene in 125 plants out of the 400 analysed (Fig 3). These 125 PCR putative positive plants and 16 more healthy looking plants from a total of 19 primary transformants were further analysed for the efficacy of the gene.

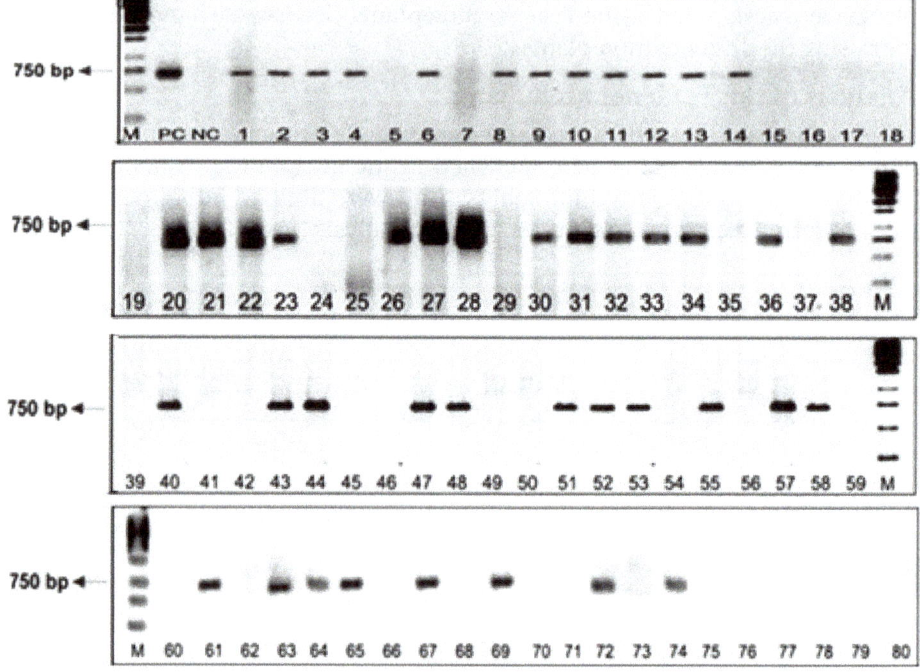

Fig 3: Grid PCR analysis of putative T_1 *cry*1X transgenic groundnut plants using *npt*II primers.

Lanes:

1-80 - Composite samples from GRID 1 to 4

M - 1kb marker

NC - Negative control

PC - Positive control (plasmid pBinBt8 DNA)

Genomic DNA was extracted from the composite leaf samples of putative T_1 groundnut transformants and PCR analysis was done using *npt*II primers to screen the transgenic plants.

Insect Resistance of the Transgenic Plants

The efficacy of the *cry* gene product was tested against two major pests of groundnut viz., *H. armigera* and *S. litura*. Leaves from 4-6 week old groundnut plants, that were positive from grid PCR analysis, were taken for bioassay. Ten neonate larvae were loaded per leaf and were monitored for 96 h. Mortality and per cent leaf damage were recorded to asses the effect of the protein on the larvae. Concurrent bioassays were also run on wild type plants. The transgenic plants showed significantly higher tolerance to the target pests and performed better when compared to the wild type (Fig 4a & 4b).

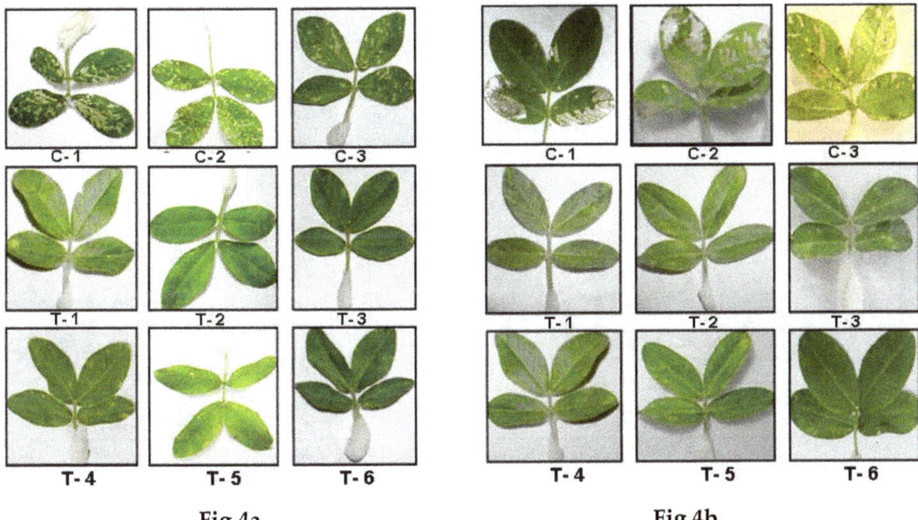

Fig 4a. Fig 4b.

Fig 4a: Leaf bioassay against *Helicoverpa armigera* larvae conducted at the laboratory. Per cent leaf area damaged by the larvae in the bioassay of groundnut control (C-1 to C-3) and putative transgenics (T-1 to T-6) transformed with cry1X gene in T1 generation.

Fig 4b: Leaf bioassay against neonate *Spodoptera litura* larvae conducted at the laboratory. Per cent leaf area damaged by the larvae in the bioassay of groundnut control (C-1 to C-3) and putative transgenics (T-1 to T-6) transformed with cry1Xgene in T1 generation.

Bioefficacy of the transgenics was assessed against the larvae of *Helicoverpa armigera* and *Spodoptera litura*. The larval mortality and damage to the leaves was recorded for a period of 96 h.

The larvae that survived after feeding on the transgenic plants were severely stunted when compared to the larvae that fed on the leaves from wild type plants in both the bioassays (Fig 5a & 5b).

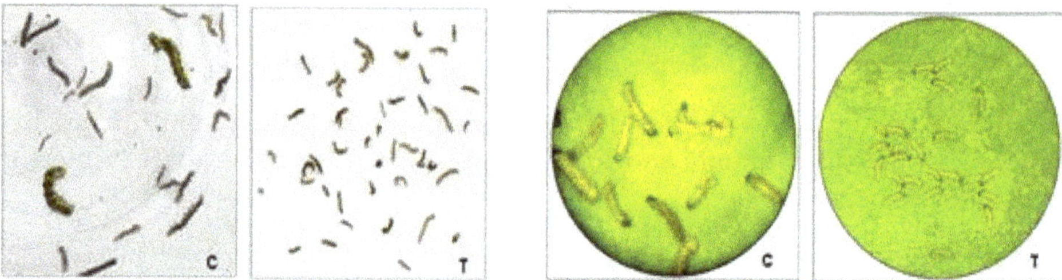

Fig 5a. **Fig 5b.**

Fig 5a: *Helicoverpa armigera* larvae fed on control (C)) and T2 transgenics (T) transformed with cry1X gene.

Fig 5b: *Spodoptera lutura* larvae fed on control (C)) and T2 transgenics (T) transformed with cry1X gene.

The strong correlation between two parameters per cent mortality and per cent damage against *Helicoverpa armigera* and *Spodoptera litura* was found (Fig 6a & 6b).

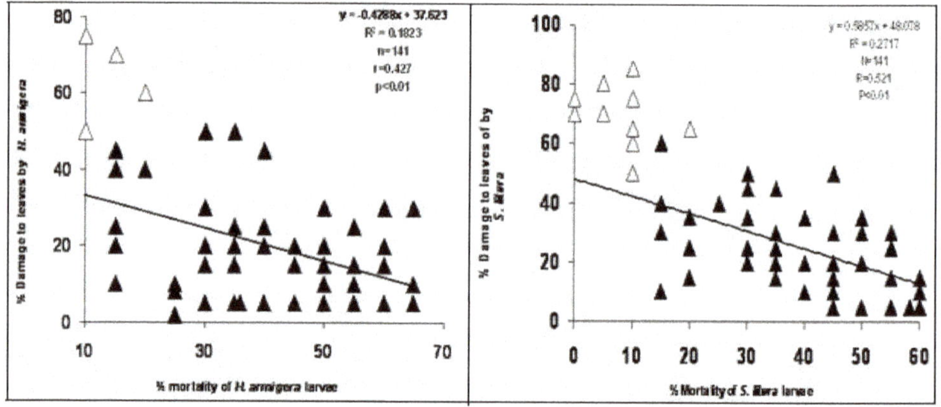

Fig 6a. **Fig 6b.**

Fig 6a: Relation between per cent mortality of neonate *Helicoverpa armigera* and per cent damage by larvae in bioassay of detached leaves of selected putative transgenic plants of T_1 generation evaluated under laboratory conditions. The relationship indicated is only for the transgenic plants and the hollow triangles represent the data for control plants.

Fig 6b: Relation between per cent mortality of neonate *Spodoptera litura* and per cent damage by larvae in bioassay of detached leaves of selected putative transgenic plants of T_1 generation evaluated under laboratory conditions. The relationship indicated is only for the transgenic plants and the hollow triangles represent the data for control plants.

Interestingly the efficacy of the chimeric gene appeared similar against both the larvae as confirmed by the strong correlation between the per cent mortalities of the two larvae by plants ($r= -0.754$; $p<0.01$; $n=141$; Fig 7a) and per cent damages to leaves caused by the two larvae ($r= 0.851$; $p<0.01$; $n=141$; Fig 7b).

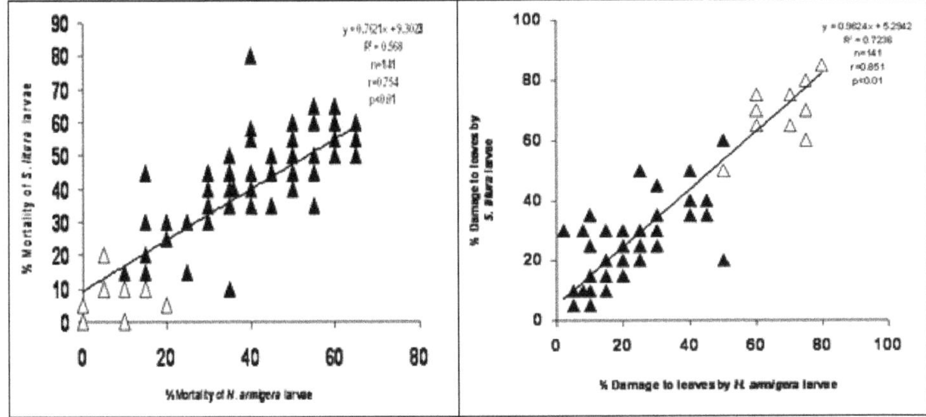

Fig 7a. **Fig 7b.**

Fig 7: Relation between the performance of neonate larvae of *Helicoverpa armigera* and *Spodoptera litura* in bioassays of detached leaves of selected putative transgenic plants of T1 generation with respect to

(a) per cent mortalities of the two larvae and
(b) per cent leaf damages by the two larvae.

The relationship indicated is only for the transgenic plants and the hollow triangles represent the data for control plants.

However, the results suggested a variable response of the transgenics towards the two larvae and a large many transgenics were found superior to wild type plants. Results of the experiments revealed that the 141 transgenic plants showed a range of 10-80 per cent mortality and 5-60 per cent damage in both the bioassays in contrast to 1-10 per cent mortality and 60-70 per cent damage in the wild type leaves. This clearly indicated the variable expression of the transferred *Bt*-gene and a consequent variable effectiveness against the target insects.

Based on the bioassays against *H. armigera* and *S. litura,* 27 plants that showed > 50 per cent mortality and not more than 10 per cent damage were selected to be taken further. Comparison of means by two tailed 't' test with unequal sample sizes, indicated the selected transgenic plants to be significantly superior to wild type plants in respect of per cent mortalities of both *H. armigera* (t = 18.01 ; p< 0.01) and *S. litura* (t = 14.67 ; p< 0.01). Similarly, the two plants differed significantly in respect of damage to leaf by both *H. armigera* (t = 17.94; p< 0.01) and *S. litura* (t = 20.14; p< 0.01) (Table 1).

Table 1: Bioefficacy of *cry*1X transgenics against *Helicoverpa armigera* and *Spodoptera litura* larvae in T_1 generation.

Treatment	T. No.	Leaf bioassay against *Helicoverpa armigera*		Leaf bioassay against *Spodoptera litura*	
		Mean ± SD		Mean ± SD	
		% Mortality	% Damage	% Mortality	% Damage
Transgenic plants	27	51.52 ± 9.42	6.11 ± 2.12	52.41 ± 8.36	5.74 ± 1.81

Treatment	T. No.	Leaf bioassay against *Helicoverpa armigera*		Leaf bioassay against *Spodoptera litura*	
		Mean ± SD		Mean ± SD	
		% Mortality	% Damage	% Mortality	% Damage
Wild type Control (Non- transgenic plants	10	8.00 ± 6.00	67.50 ± 9.01	8.00 ± 5.57	69.50 ± 9.60
't'- test					
't'		18.012	17.945	14.686	20.146
probability		p<0.01	p<0.01	p<0.01	p<0.01

p<0.01, significance at 1% level.

The T_1 transgenics were analysed for bioefficacy by leaf bioassay against *Helicoverpa armigera* and *Spodoptera litura*. The range in per cent mortality and per cent damage are given in the table.

Confirmation of the integration and inheritance of the transgene in all 27 selected plants was obtained by PCR analysis for *npt*II and *cry*1X gene. Results show amplification at 750 bp for *npt*II gene and 950 bp for *cry*1X gene (Fig 8a & 8b).

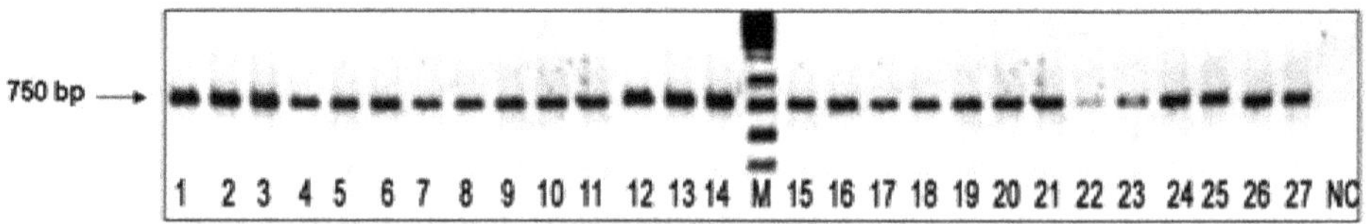

Fig 8a: PCR analysis of the T_1 transgenics expressing *npt*II gene.

Lanes:	
1-27	- DNA from the transgenic plants
M	- 1kb marker
NC	- Negative control
PC	- Positive control (plasmid **pBinBt8** DNA)

Genomic DNA was extracted from the leaf samples of putative T_1 groundnut transformants and PCR analysis was done using primers for *np*II gene to screen the transgenic plants.

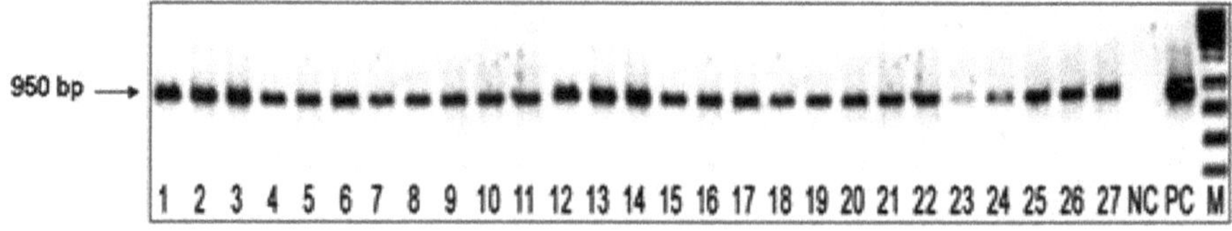

Fig 8b: PCR analysis of the T_2 transgenics expressing *cry*1X gene.

Lanes:

1-27	-	DNA from the transgenic plants
M	-	1kb marker
NC	-	Negative control
PC	-	Positive control (plasmid pBinBt8 DNA)

Genomic DNA was extracted from the composite leaf samples of putative T_2 cotton transformants and PCR analysis was done using gene specific primers (*cry*1X) to screen the transgenic plants.

Therefore, the 27 plants thus confirmed as transgenics based on PCR and bioassays against *H. armigera and S. litura,* were selected for further advancement.

Analysis of the T_2 Generation Groundnut Plants Harboring the *cry* 1X gene

The seeds of the 27 best transgenics proved in T_1 generation were sown in the greenhouse. Of these, 340 plants could be obtained. The transgenics (340 plants) that were germinated in T_2 generation was subjected to PCR by using primers for *npt*II gene. Results show amplification at 750 bp in 322 plants (Fig 9a & 9b).

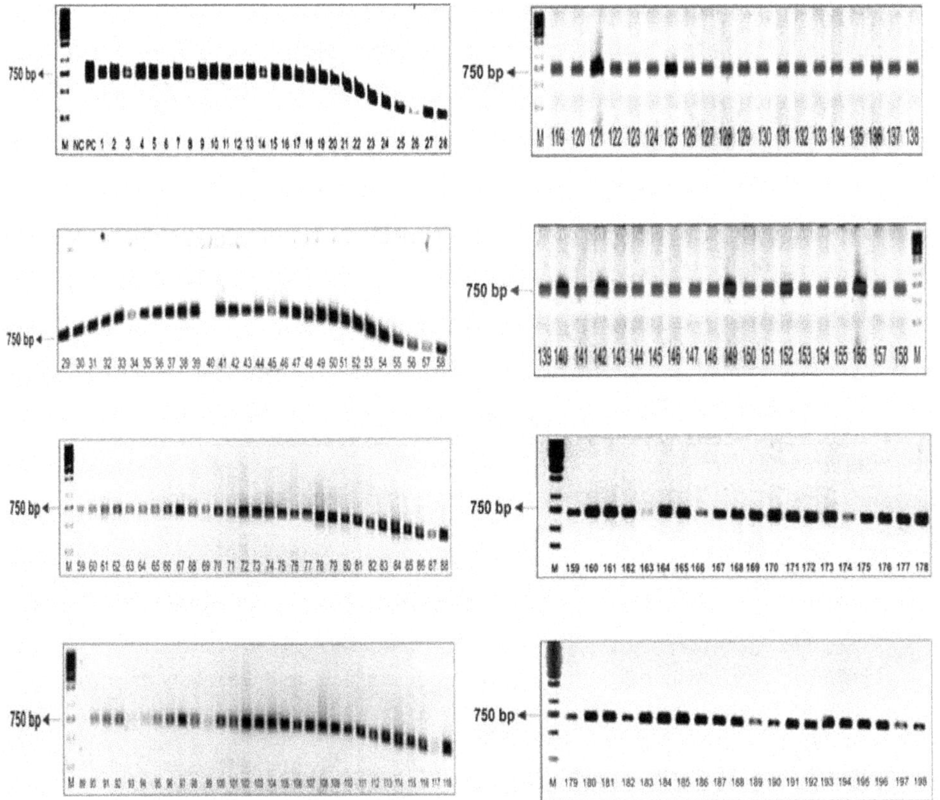

Fig 9a: PCR analysis of the T_2 transgenics using *npt*II primers.

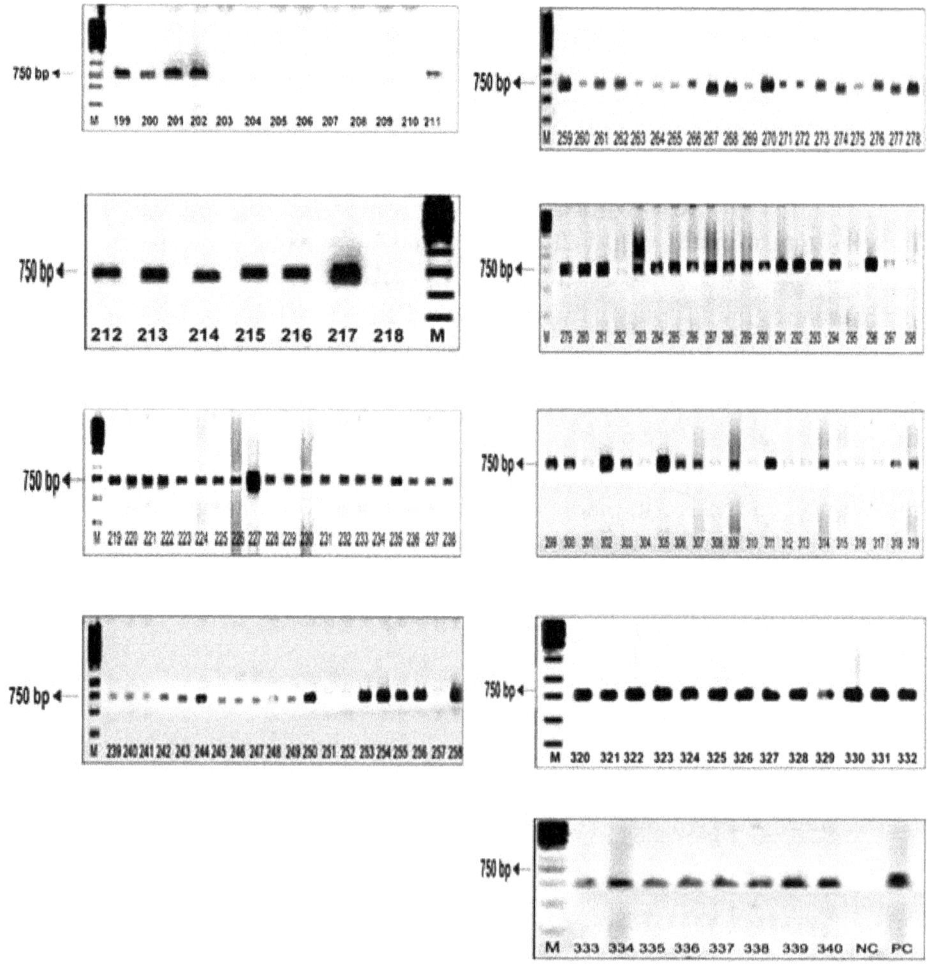

Fig 9b: PCR analysis of the T_2 transgenics using *npt*II primer.

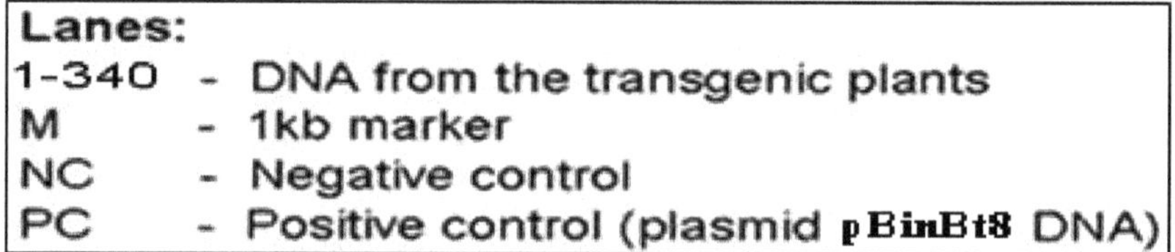

Lanes:

1-340	-	DNA from the transgenic plants
M	-	1kb marker
NC	-	Negative control
PC	-	Positive control (plasmid **pBinBt8** DNA)

Genomic DNA was extracted from the composite leaf samples of putative T_2 ground transformants and PCR analysis was done using *npt*II primers to screen the transgenic plants.

Further, when all the 340 plants were subjected to ELISA, high expression was observed in 90 plants, showing 3-16 fold increase over the negative control (Fig 10).

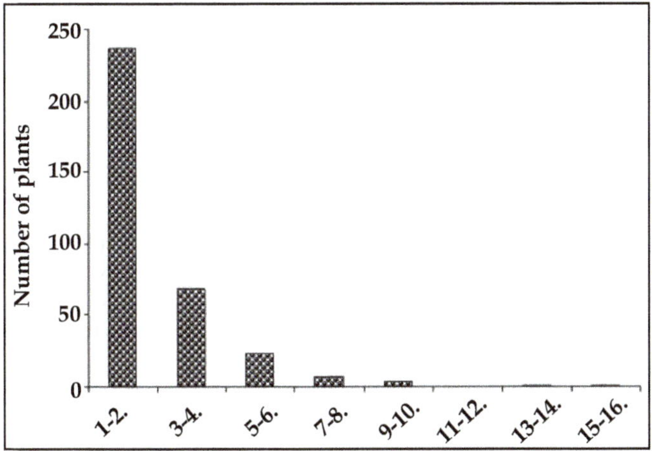

Fig 10: Frequency distribution of putative transgenics transformed with *cry*1X gene for fold increase in ELISA values of transgenics over the negative control among 340 plants of groundnut in T_2 generation.

Analysis of 10 high expressing plants from T2 generation (Fig 11 (a) to 11 (e). High expressing plants based on ELISA (10 plants that showed 7-16 fold increase over the negative control) (Fig 11a) were selected for molecular characterization by PCR and genomic Southern analysis. A 950 bp *cry*1X fragment was amplified in all the 10 plants suggesting stability and integration (Fig 11b) and strip test (the arrow shows expression (Fig 11c). These plants were subjected to genomic Southern analysis. High molecular weight uncut DNA hybridized with the 950 bp random prime labeled *cry*1X gene fragment revealing integration of transgene (Fig 11d). In the vector used for raising the transgenic plants, *Bam*HI releases a 1.9 kb fragment which includes the *cry*1X gene. The hybridization signal at the right position indicates (Fig 11e) the integration of the transgene.

Howeer, the 15 best lines was selected for further advancement from T_2 generation.

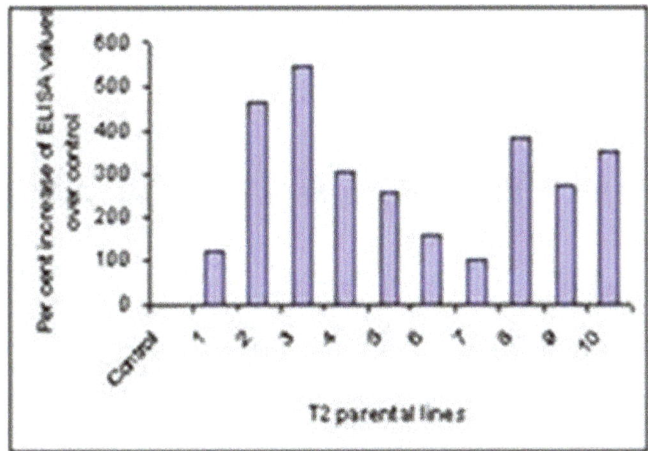

Fig 11 (a): ELISA for *cry*1X expression - fold increase in ELISA values of selected 10 transgenics over the negative control.

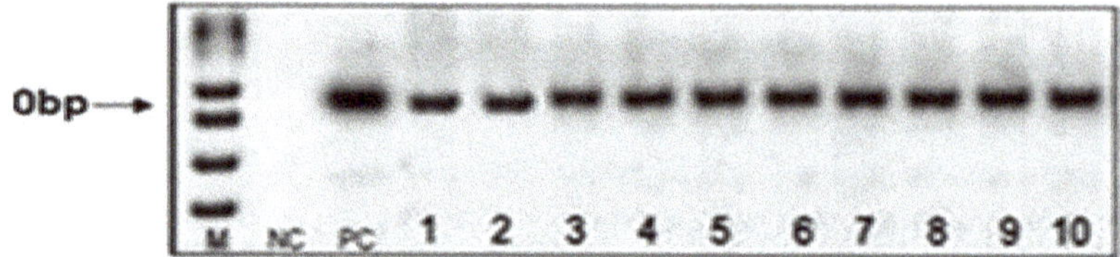

Fig 11 (b): PCR of the DNA of transgenic plants transformed with *cry*1X gene in the T_2 generation groundnut using primers for *cry*1X gene. Lane M: DNA ladder (1 kb); Lane NC: negative control (DNA from untransformed plants); Lane PC: positive control (plasmid pBinBt8 DNA); Lanes 1-10: DNA from putative transformants.

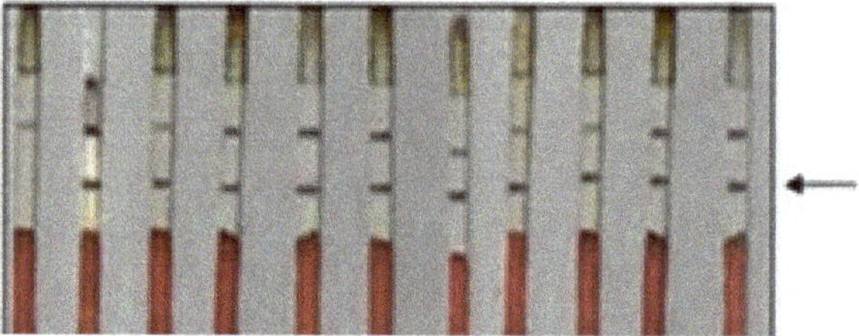

Fig 11 (c): Quickstix showing the protein band at the expected position (arrow marked) identifying the chimeric *Bt* protein in 10 plants and absence in the control.

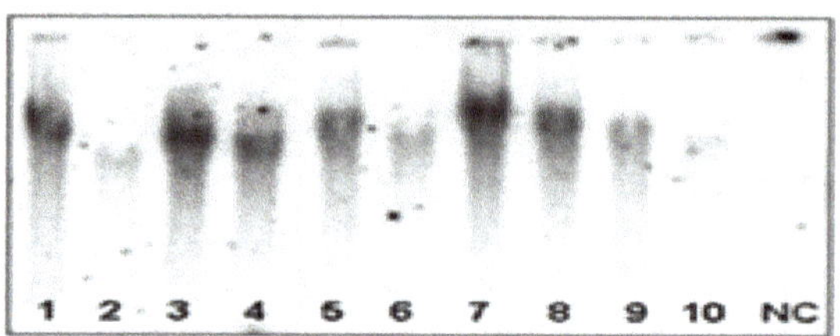

Fig 11 (d): Southern hybridization of uncut DNA of T_2 transformants probed with radiolabelled 950 bp of *cry*1X gene. Lanes 1-10: DNA from putative transformants; Lane NC: Negative control (DNA from untransformed plants).

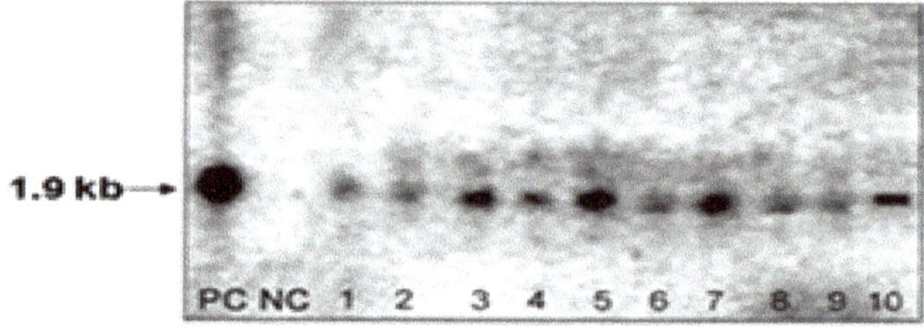

Fig 11 (e): Southern hybridization of DNA of T_2 transformants digested with *Bam*HI and probed with radiolabelled 950 bp product of *cry*1X gene. Lane NC: Negative control (DNA from untransformed plants); Lane PC: Positive control (plasmid pBinBt8 DNA); Lanes 1-10: DNA from putative transformants.

Discussion

The successful cultivation of bollworm resistant *Bt* cotton varieties has provided a great impetus for the development of a large number of transgenics that are potentially capable of alleviating many pest and disease problems in different crops. Engineering for insect pest resistance in legumes (Sharma *et al.*, 2006, Ignacimuthu *et al.*, 2006) is being considered important in the recent years. However, very little progress is seen in the improvement of legumes through transgenic approach and more so with groundnut because of the recalcitrancy in regeneration of the crop. There are reports of regenerability in groundnut, but with less frequency, using leaf discs and leaf section explants (Eapen and George 1994, Cheng *et al.*, 1996), cotyledons (Venkatachalam *et al.*, 2000, Bhatnagar *et al.*, 2007), cotyledonary node (Anuradha *et al.*, 2006). Recalcitrance and genotype-dependent regeneration called for standardization of alternate methods of transformation that totally avoid tissue culture and consequent regeneration needs that is often genotype dependent (Rohini and Sankara Rao, 2000a, 2000b and 2001). The methodology is therefore, readily available for adoption in the transformation of groundnut with relatively higher expectations of success. Nevertheless, very less progress has been made with improvement of Indian cultivars of groundnut with respect to insect pest resistance using transgenic technology. This work reports the successful transformation of groundnut cv. TMV-2 for insect pest resistance using a chimeric *cry* gene, *cry*1X.

The method is based on the fact that some of the differentiated embryonic cells that take in the DNA can develop into germ cells and therefore will be transmitted to the next generation. The meristem transformation protocols are being used as *in planta* transformation protocols for the improvement of difficult-to-regenerate species (Sankara Rao and Rohini 1999, Rohini and Sankara Rao, 2000a, 2000b and 2001. Earlier, chitinase gene for fungal disease resistance was introduced into groundnut using the *in planta* transformation protocol demonstrating the feasibility of this protocol to develop stable transformants (Rohini and Sankara Rao, 2000a and 2000b).

In our method, *A. tumefaciens* is targeted to the wounded apical meristem of the differentiated seed embryo. Therefore, *A. tumefaciens* transfers the gene into the genome of diverse cells which are already destined to develop into specific organs and the meristematic cells still to be differentiated. This results in the primary transformants (T_0) being chimeric in nature. Consequently, this necessitates the analysis of the putative transgenic plants only in the T_1 generation. The chimeric plants producing the transformants in the T_1 generation depends on the type of cells that were transformed in the T_0 plants. If the transgene is integrated into undifferentiated meristematic cells that are destined to develop into branches, seeds obtained from the reproductive structures of these branches are expected to give stable transformants in T_1. The *in planta* transformation protocol gives rise to a large number of T_1 generation plants and a preliminary screening procedure is required that considerably reduces the number of putative transformants to be taken forward. Grid PCR technique helps eliminate many plants by using composite DNA samples in a PCR reaction. While all plants eliminated are truly non-transformants, the methodology, does not help identify the putative transformants, as the selected plants are a mixture of both non-transformants and the transformants. Therefore, the plants contributing for a positive composite sample in the grid PCR have to be further checked to identify the individual putative transgenics. Hence, grid PCR positive composite samples were taken ahead for further analysis. Initially insect reactions against two target pests viz., *H. armigera* and *S. litura* based on bioassays were assessed and subsequently the resistant lines were further analysed for integration and expression.

Development of transgenic crops being a long lasting and high investment option a major threat for the long lasting effect of such crops is the potentiality of the insects to develop resistance against such crops. Therefore, it is envisaged that gene pyramiding in transgenic plants could be a potentially more viable strategy for delaying the insect pest evolution leading to resistance against single *cry* genes (Cao *et al.,* 2002, Greenplate *et al.,* 2000). It is also expected that the same option might also help improve the efficacy range of the introduced genes covering more than one or a set of species (Datta *et al.,* 2002a). An alternative to the gene pyramiding would be to use synthetic genes of multiple efficacies. Earlier studies in transgenic potato with *cry*1Ba/*cry*11a hybrid gene encoding a protein consisting of domains I and III of *cry1Ba* and domain II of *cry*1Ia demonstrated resistance against both Coleoptera represented by colorado potato beetle larvae and adults and Lepidoptera represented by potato tuber moth larvae and european corn borer larvae.

Similar results were anticipated from our selection of the *cry*1X gene in the present study. The chimeric *cry* gene, *cry*1X, has domains from four *cry* genes, *cry*1Ac, *cry*1Ab, *cry*1Aa3 and *cry*1F. *Cry*1Ac, Ab, and Aa3 are effective against *H. armigera* whereas, *cry*1F is best against *S. litura*. Thus it was anticipated that the novel construct would provide protection against at least two entirely differing groups of Lepidopteran pests with different *Bt* protoxin receptors. Further, due to the fact that the gene encodes the active domains of four different *Bt* toxins, it is anticipated that it might work against a far diverse species of Lepidoptera. These expectations were substantiated by the fact that the efficacy of the *cry*1Xgene was confirmed, albeit variable, in bioassays against *H. armigera* and *S. litura*.

There were significant differences between the per cent mortality in the transgenics when compared to those of non-transgenic wild types indicating the effectiveness of the *Bt* toxin in the transgenics. The pattern repeated with both the species.

The observed mortality patterns of both the target pests in T_1 generation clearly suggested the variable expression levels of the transgene in this generation. Further, the range of the variability being sufficiently large, the mortality data was regressed against the leaf damage. It was observed that the mortality was strongly negatively correlated with the extent of leaf damage when groundnut leaves were challenged with neonates of *H. armigera* or *S. litura*. Clearly, these results indicate that the mortality of the larvae is a product of the extent of ingestion of toxin that was inversely related to the total food consumed. Thus the plants with low levels of expression of the transgene experienced greater extent of leaf loss and resulted in better survival of the larvae. More interestingly, the toxin appeared to be equally effective at levels of expression against the two larvae of disparate *Bt* toxin protoxin receptors, as the mortality levels of the two larvae against the plants were strongly and positively correlated. Further, 27 plants that had high per cent mortality and per cent damage were selected and continued into the next generation and analyzed for the stability of the transgene. These plants showed mortality in a range of 40-80 per cent and damage as low as 5-10 per cent which corroborated in the bioassays against both *Helicoverpa armigera* and *Spodoptera litura.*

In the progeny of these 27 plants in the T_2 generation, 322 plants out of 340 plants developed in the greenhouse were PCR positives suggesting segregation in some of the lines. However, 90 plants showed very high ELISA values and there was variation between the transgenic plants when compared to the wild type. Such variations in protein expression levels in different transgenic bioassays are quite frequent and common due to genotypic, developmental and environmental control. Such variations have also been observed among the progenies of a single parental line with an identical pattern of transgene integration and grown under the same environment (Datta *et al.*, 1998, Aguda *et al.*, 2001, Alinia *et al.*, 2001, Datta *et al.*, 2002a,Marfa *et al.*, 2002). To confirm the integration of the transgene in the groundnut plants (T_2 generation) showing high ELISA values, genomic southern analysis was performed with the DNA of 10 plants that showed high expression. Strips test carried out in the plants selected for southern analysis supported the ELISA data. Hybridization of uncut DNA and release of 1.9 kb fragment after digestion with *Bam*HI and a strong hybridization signal after probing with a radiolabelled PCR product of the *cry*1Xgene clearly demonstrated integration, inheritance and stability of the transgene. Nevertheless, copy number studies needs to be carried out to select and take further the events with single copy insertions of the gene.

Transformation efficiency in the present study was calculated using per cent mortality of *Helicoverpa armigera* as a parameter. Among the individual transformants exhibiting >3σ (SD) of the wild type plants (SD= 6.32), 63.12% of the total 141 transformants showed higher values with a mean value of 42.42. This resulted in 88 plants performing well which is 22% of the 400 plants taken for T_1 analysis. These plants can be considered as putative transformants. However, 27 plants which showed mortality of >56% were selected for further analysis into the next generation and were subsequently confirmed as transgenics by molecular analysis. This study presents the following, (1) evidence for the production of insect resistant plants using the *in planta* transformation protocol. (2) efficacy of the chimeric *Bt*-gene against Lepidopteran pests, *Helicoverpa armigera* and *Spodoptera litura,* two major leaf eating caterpillars of groundnut. The successful advancement of these transgenics containing the *cry*1X gene in groundnut to obtain the stable lines will provide a seed borne solution to manage some Lepidopteran pest of groundnut.

Summary

Insects pose a perennial problem to crops. Yield reductions are mainly due to insect damage. The important pests that have become a constraint are the pod/ boll borers *Helicoverpa armigera* and the leaf-eating caterpillars like *Spodoptera litura* and *Amsacta albistriga* (RHHC). Breeding for resistance against these pests is a potential option. However, alternate source becomes a pre-requisite as there are no resistant sources available to these pests. This apparently calls for the use of genetic engineering techniques to produce insect tolerant crops by gene transfer technology, using effective genes.

Methods that avoid tissue culture steps or the *in planta* transformation strategy could be a viable option. The transgenic plant recovery achieved in this study was by a tissue culture-independent method (Sankara Rao and Rohini, 1999; Rohini and Sankara Rao, 2000a, 2000b and 2001) *i.e.*, by germination of the *Agrobacterium*-treated embryo from a mature seed. The possibility of developing stable transformants by *in planta* transformation technique has been demonstrated in several other crops like buckwheat (Kojima *et al.*, 2000), mulberry (Ping *et al.*, 2003), kenaf (Kojima *et al.*, 2004), rice (Supartana *et al.*, 2005), wheat (Supartana *et al.*, 2006) and maize (Chumakov *et al.*, 2006), apart from *Arabidopsis thaliana* (Feldman and Marks, 1987) and soybean (Chee *et al.*, 1989).

The development of a viable transgenic crop plant depends on the availability of a gene of choice, a suitable delivery system for the insertion of the gene and the methodology of selecting the best possible transformants. A large variety of genes in the *cry* family of *Bt* delta-endotoxins such as *cry*1Ab, *cry*1Ac, *cry*2Aa, *cry*2Ab, and *Vip*3A are known to be effective against *Helicoverpa armigera* and many have already been used successfully for development of resistant transgenics. Further several methods to deliver genes into plant system have been developed. But yet all the methods are not equally amenable for use with all the crops. Most economically important plants are recalcitrant and not amenable to tissue culture regeneration. Therefore, there is a need to adopt plant transformation methods that exclude tissue culture steps and rely on alternate protocols for the transformation of such recalcitrant crop plants.

It is now firmly established that transgenics are bound to become the mainstay of the pest management technology in the years to come. However, the role of insect pests in limiting the productivity of crops is of no less importance in the marginalized crops and agri-ecosystems. Dry land crops are generally low input crops in the first place and next, due to eccentricity of monsoon, risk associated with further investment can be very high and can be a potential perennial problem. As a result, seed borne solutions at meaningful cost prices would facilitate better performance of the crops against insect pests.

Besides molecular characterization of the transgenics, expression analysis and bioefficacy assessment of the transformants is crucial for the superior event. Therefore the major focus of this study was to,

1. Develop an efficient *in planta* transformation protocol in groundnut at nano levels.

2. Generate transformants in groundnut for expressing a novel *cry* gene, *cry*1X.
3. Molecular and bioefficacy characterization of transgenics expressing *cry*1X to identify stable and high efficacy lines.

To achieve this, we selected a chimeric *cry* gene with domains from four different *cry* genes which would provide broad spectrum resistance towards many insects. We adapted *in planta* transformation technique to develop transformants and using diverse tools we characterized T_1 and the subsequent generations for integration, expression and efficacy. Ultimately, our aim has been to identify stable transformants expressing *cry*1X which would show resistance against *Helicoverpa* and *Spodoptera.*

Analysis of the Groundnut Transformants for High Expressing Lines Against Insect Pests

Grid PCR analysis was carried out with 400 T_1 plants raised from 25 T_0 plants. Among them, 125 putative transformants were checked for bioefficacy against two insect pests of groundnut viz., *Helicoverpa armigera* and *Spodoptera litura.* Bioassays followed by PCR for the amplification of the *cry* gene resulted in the selection of 27 plants for analysis into the next generation. In the analysis of T_2 generation plants, 340 plants were first analysed by PCR and 90 high expressing lines were selected based on ELISA. Nevertheless, 15 plants from 9 T_1 background were selected for further analysis.

PCR analysis of the grid samples was the first analysis in the T_1 generation. Grid PCR positive composite samples were taken ahead for further analysis against insects. Initially insect reactions against two target pests viz., *H. armigera* and *S. litura* based on bioassays were assessed and subsequently the resistant lines were further analyzed for integration and expression. There were significant differences between the per cent mortality in the transgenics when compared to those of non-transgenic wild types indicating the effectiveness of the *Bt* toxin in the transgenics. The pattern repeated with both the species. The observed mortality patterns of both the target pests in the T_1 generation clearly suggested the variable expression levels of the transgene in this generation. Further, the range of the variability being sufficiently large, the mortality data was regressed against leaf damage. It was observed that the mortality was strongly negatively correlated with the extent of leaf damage when groundnut leaves were challenged with neonates of *H. armigera* or *S. litura.* Clearly, these results indicate that the mortality of the larvae is a product of the extent of ingestion of toxin that was inversely related to the total food consumed. Thus the plants with low levels of expression of the transgene experienced greater extent of leaf loss and resulted in better survival of the larvae. More interestingly, the toxin appeared to be equally effective at levels of expression against the two larvae of disparate *Bt* toxin protoxin receptors, as the mortality levels of the two larvae against the plants were strongly and positively correlated. Further, the 27 plants that had a high per cent mortality and per cent damage were selected and continued into the next generation and analyzed for the stability of the transgene. These plants showed mortality in a range of 40-80 per cent and damage as low as 5-10 per cent which corroborated in the bioassays against both *Helicoverpa armigera* and *Spodoptera litura*.

In the progeny of these 27 plants in the T_2 generation, 322 plants out of 340 plants developed in the greenhouse were PCR positives suggesting segregation in some of the lines. However, 90 plants showed very high ELISA values and there was variation between the transgenic plants when compared to the wild type.

Strips test carried out in the plants selected for southern analysis supported the ELISA data. Hybridization of uncut DNA and the release of a 1.9 kb fragment after digestion with *Bam*HI and a strong hybridization signal after probing with a radiolabelled PCR product for the *cry*1Xgene clearly demonstrated integration, inheritance and stability of the transgene. Nevertheless, copy number studies need to be carried out to select and take further the events with single copy insertions of the gene.

The study although is only a preliminary one, substantially suggests the possibility of developing efficient *cry* gene harboring transgenics that can provide good protection against the major pests of field bean, cotton and groundnut. The study overwhelmingly demonstrated the following,

(a) Effective *cry* genes that can work against the major pests of field bean, cotton and groundnut exist.

(b) *In planta* method can provide viable field bean, cotton and groundnut transformants against insect pests.

(c) Over expression of *cry* genes provides reasonably good resistance against pod borers especially, *Helicoverpa armigera* and *Spodoptera litura*.

(d) Some of the promising lines were identified in all the three species and few commercially viable events can be developed after field evaluation.

Future Line of Work

The selected plants based on the integration, expression and efficacy of the *cry*1X gene in groundnut crops has to be evaluated further for the site of integration of the transgene and subsequently generate event specific molecular information. Further advancement of the selected lines to assess their performance under field conditions.

References

Aguda RM., Datta K., Tu SK., Datta., Cohen MB.,(2001). Expression of *Bt* genes under control of different promoters in rice at vegetative and flowering stages. *Int Rice Res*. Notes, 26 : 26-27.

Alinia FB., Ghareyazio., Rubia J., Bennett., Cohen MB., (2001). Expression of effect of plant age, larval age, and fertilizer treatment on resistance of a *cry*1Ab-transformed aromatic rice to Lepidopterans stem borers and foliage feeders. *J. Econ. Entomol*,93 : 484-493.

Azipiroz-Leehan R and Feldmann KA.,(1997)T-DNA insertion mutagenesis in *Arabidopsis* : going back and forth, *Trends Gene.*13, 152-156.

Bechtold N., Ellis J., Pelletier G., (1993). *In plantaAgrobacterium*-mediated gene transfer by infiltration of adult *Arabidopsis thaliana* plants. *C.R Acad Sci Paris Life Sci*,316 : 1194-1199.

BhatnagarMathur P., Devi MJ., Reddy DS., Lavanya M., Vadez V., Serraj R., YamaguchiShinozaki K., Sharma KK., (2007). Stress induced expression of *At* DREB1A in transgenic peanut (*Arachis hypogaea* L.) increases transcription efficiency under water – limiting conditions. *Plant Cell Rep* (online version).

Brahmaprakash G P., Chandraprakash J., Ganeshaiah K N. and Uma Shankar R., (2004). Pulse yields, Feeling the pulse, *Current Science.* 87 (7) : 859 - 861.

Cao J., Zhao JZ., Shelton AM., Earle ED., (2002). Broccoli plants pyramided with *cry*1AC and *cry*1C *Bt* gene control diamondback moths resistance to *cry*1A and *cry*1AC proteins. *Theor. Appl. Genet*,105 : 258-264.

Cheng M., Jarret RL., Li Z and Xing JW., (1996). Demski, Production of fertile transgenic peanut (*Arachis hypogeae* L.) plants using *Agrobacterium ttumefaciens.Plant Cell Rep*, 15 : 653-657.

Datta K., Baisakh N., Thet KM., Tu J., Datta SK., (2002a). Pyramiding transgenes for multiple resistance in rice against bacterial blight, stem borer and sheath blight. *Theor. Appl. Genet*,106 : 1-8.

Datta K., Varquez A., Tu J., Torrizo L., Alam MF., Oliva N., Abrigo E., Khush GS and Datta SK., (1998). Constitutive and tissue specific differential expression of *cry*1A(b*)* gene in transgenic rice plants conferring enhanced resistance to insect pests. *Theor. Appl. Genet*, 97 : 20-30.

Dellaporta S L., Wood J and Hicks J B., (1983). A plant DNA minipreparation : version II. *Plant Mol Biol Rep*, 1 : 19-21.

Eapen S., George L., (1994). *Agrobacterium tumefaciens* mediated gene transfer in peanut (*Arachis hypogaea* L.). *Plant Cell Rep*,13 : 582-586.

Greenplate JT., Penn SR., Shappley Z., Oppenhuizen M., Mann J., Reich B and Oshorn J., (2000). Bollgard II efficacy : Quantification of total Lepidopteran activity in a two gene product. *Proc. Belt wide cotton conf*,2 : 1041-1043.

Ignacimuthu S., Prakash S., (2006). *Agrobacterium*-mediated transformation of chickpea with α-amylase inhibitor gene for insect resistance. *Journal of Biosciences*,31(3) : 339-345.

Keshamma E., Rohini Sreevathsa., Manoj Kumar A., Kalpana N Reddy., Manjulatha M., Shanmugam N B., Kumar A R V and Udayakumar M., (2012). *Agrobacterium*-Mediated *in Planta* Transformation of Field Bean (*Lablab Purpureus* L.) and Recovery of Stable Transgenic Plants Expressing the *cry*1AcF Gene. Plant Mol. Biol. Rep. (DOI 10.1007/s11105-011-0312-7). Published online: 12 May 2011. Released on Februaary 2012, Volume 30, issue 1, pp 67-78. (Springer Publication).

Keshamma K., Rohini S., Madhusudhan B and Prasad T G., (2008). Transformability in Field bean (*uid* A :: *npt* II) by *Agrobacterium tumefaciens* - mediated *in planta* strategy. J Plant Biol. Vol. 35 (1), pp. 31-37. (Society for Plant Physiology and Biochemistry).

Liao C., Heckle D G., Akhrust R., (2002). Toxicity of Bacillus thuringiensis insecticidal proteins for *Helicoverpa armigera* and *Helicoverpa punctigera* (Lepidoptera : Noctuidae), major pests of cotton. *Journal of Invertebrate Pathology*, 80 : 55 - 63.

Marfa V., Mele E., Gabarra R., Vassal JM., Guiderdoni E., Messeguer J., (2002). Influence of the development stage of transgenic rice plants (cv. Senia) expressing the *cry*1B gene on the level of protection against the striped stem borer (*Chilo suppressalis*). *Plant cell Rep,* 20 : 1167-1172.

Rohini and Sankara Rao., (1999). Gene transfer into Indian cultivars of Safflower (*Carthamus tinctorium* L.) using *Agrobacteriu tumefaciens*. *Plant Biotechnology,* **16 (3)** : 201-206.

Rohini and Sankara Rao., (2000a). Embryo transformation, a practical approach for realizing transgenic plants of safflower (*Carthamus tinctorius* L.). *Ann. Bot,* 86 : 1043-1049.

Rohini and Sankara Rao., (2001). Transformation of peanut (*Arachis hypogaea* L.) with tobacco chitinase gene : variable response of transformants to leaf spot disease. *Plant Science,*160 (5) : 883-892.

Rohini and Sankara Rao., (2000b). Transformation of peanut (*Arachis hypogaea* L.): a non-tissue culture based approach for generating transgenic plants. *Plant Science,*150 : 41-49.

Sambrook J., Fritsch EF and Maniatis T., (1989). Molecular cloning, Plain view, New York, Cold Spring Harbor Laboratory Press.

Sankara Rao K., Rohini Sreevasthsa., Keshamma E and Udaya Kumar M.,(2008). *In planta* transformation of pigeon pea : a method to overcome recalcitrance of the crop to regeneration *in vitro*. *Physiol. Mol. Plants*. 14 (4) : 321-328.

Sharma KK., Lavanya M., Anjaiah., (2006). *Agrobacterium* mediated production of transgenic pigeonpea (*Cajanus cajan* L.Milisp.) expressing the synthetic *Bt cry*1Ab gene. *In vitro Cell. Dev. Biol.-Plant,*42 : 165-173.

Snedecor G and Cochran WG., (1967). Statistical methods. Oxford and IBH Publishing Co. pp. 593.

Sokal RR and Rohlf FJ., (1969). Biometry : the principles and practices of statistics in biological research. Freeman W.H and Co., San Francisco : 776 p.

Sundaresha S., Rohini S., MathSA., Keshamma E., Chandrashekar SC., Udaya Kumar M., (2010). Enhanced protection against two major fungus pathogens of groundnut, *Cercospora arachidicola* and *Aspergillus flavus* in transgenic groundnut over expressing a tobacco B-1-3 glucanase. *Eur J Plant Pathol* 126:497-508. (Springer Publicaion)

Venkatachalam P., Geetha N., Khandelwal A., Shaila MS., Lakshmi Sita G., (2000). *Agrobacterium* mediated genetic transformation from cotyledonary explants of groundnut (*Arachis hypogaea* L.) via somatic embryogenesis. *Curr. Sci*,78 : 1130-1136.

Winans SC., Kerstetter RA and Nester EW., (1988). Transcriptional regulation of the *vir*A and *vir*G genes of *Agrobacterium tumefaciens.Journal of Bacteriology*,170 : 4047-4054.

Innovations in Biochemical Techniques (2020) : Page no. 52-64
ASTRAL INTERNATIONAL (P) LTD., New Delhi - 110002

Chapter 4

In Vitro Cytotoxicity of Silver Nanoparticles Against Human Breast Cancer (MCF-7) Cell Lines under Oxygen Limiting Conditions

B.Gowramma[1], P.G.Thejeswini[1] and Muralidhara Rao[2]

Department of Biotechnology[1], Veerashaiva College, Bellary-583104 Department of Biotechnology[2], Sri Krishnadevaraya University, Anantapuram-515003 Mail: gowriswamy6@gmail.com,

Abstract

In the present study, *in vitro* cytotoxicity activity of silver nanoparticles from *Corynebacterium glutamicum* against Human breast cancer (MCF-7) cell lines under oxygen limiting conditions has been reported. AgNPs were showing good cytotoxic effect by dose dependent manner both under normoxia and hypoxia condition. The IC_{50} values of AgNPs against MCF-7 cell lines was found to be 82.36 μg/ml under normoxia and 96.20 μg/ml under hypoxia conditions.They also inducing the Reactive Oxygen Species (ROS) and causing the cell death. From the flow cytometric studies AgNPs were showing almost 100% of apoptosis that is 99.6% of apoptosis, 0.02% of late apoptosis showing against MCF-7 cells. Hence the current investigation proves that, the Silver nanoparticles can remove the solid tumours.

Keywords: Human Breast Cancer (MCF-7) Cell Lines, Silver Nanoparticles, Normoxia, Hypoxia, Cytotoxicity

Introduction

Silver has a long history of use by humans. In ancient times it was used to purify and store water. Alexander the Great (335 BC) drank water from silver containing vessels (Russel *et al.* 1994). Besides its antimicrobial effect, AgNPs are known to induce toxicity in many different species (Bilberg *et al.*, 2011). Nanoparticles possess unique chemical, physical and biological properties, and hence it finds use in various fields like business, therapeutics, electronics, cosmetics, catalysis and drug delivery (Sriram *et al.* 2012). It offers a new view for tumor detection, prevention and treatment. Nanoparticles eradicate cancer cells by flow and penetration to different regions of tumors through blood vessels and then to interstitial space to arrive at the target cells. The environmental and physiological characteristics vary from one tumor tissues to another. Hence nanoparticles should be designed in such manner, taking into account the target site and route of administration to generate optimal therapeutic effects (Wang *et al.* 2014). Cytotoxicity studies of silver nanoparticles using plant extracts: *Melia dubia*—human breast cancer cell line (Kathiravan *et al.* 2014), *Malus domestica* (apple) extract—MCF7 (Lokina *et al.* 2014), *Inonotus obliquus* (Chaga mushroom) extract—A549 human lung cancer (CCL185) and MCF7 human breast cancer (HTB22) cell lines (Nagajyothi *et al.* 2014), *Erythrina indica*—breast and lung cancer cell lines (Rathi Sre *et al.* 2015), *Piper longum* fruit—breast cancer cell lines (Reddy *et al.* 2014), *Annona squamosa* and *Brassica Oleracea.* var. *botrytis*—MCF-7 (Ranjitham *et al.* 2013) are reported. AgNPs are cytotoxic to cancer cells and possess excellent potential as an antitumor agent, in which AgNPs induce cytotoxicity, generate reactive oxygen species (ROS), and cause mitochondrial damage to human cells. Toxic effects indifferent cell types depend on the interactions and distribution patterns of the nanoparticles .The size of nanoparticles influences the binding and activation of membrane receptors and subsequent protein expression in cancer cells (Xi Feng *et al.* 2016). Toxicological investigations of NPs imply that, *e.g.*, size, shape, chemical composition, surface charge, solubility, their ability to bind and affect biological sites as well as their metabolism and excretion influence the toxicity of NPs (Castranova, 2011).

Oxygen is the one of the limiting factor for tumor growth, tumors can withstand under oxygen limiting conditions by the help of Hypoxic Inducing Factors (HIF). Hence there is regeneration of solid tumors. The current focuses on the control of tumors under hypoxic conditions.

Materials and Method

Silver nanoparticles (Gowramma *et al.*, 2014)

Human Breast Cancer Cell Lines (MCF-7)

MCF-7 is mammary epithelial cells of breast cancer. MCF-7 cells are useful for *in vitro* breast cancer studies because the cell line has retained several ideal characteristics particular to the mammary epithelium. These include the ability for MCF-7 cells to process estrogen, in the form of estradiol, via estrogen receptors in the cell cytoplasm. This makes the MCF-7 cell line an estrogen receptor (ER) positive control cell line. In addition to retaining their estrogen sensitivity, MCF-7 cells are also sensitive to cytokeratin. They are unreceptive to desmin, endothelin, GAP, and vimentin. When grown *in vitro,* the cell line is capable of forming domes and the epithelial like cells grow in monolayers.

MCF-7 cancer cell lines were purchased from National Centre for Cell Science, Pune, India).

MCF-7 were grown in DMEM-HG supplemented with 10% heat-inactivated FBS, 2% Penicillin-Streptomycin and 2.5 µg/mL Amphotericin-B solution(All from HiMedia Labs, Mumbai, India); and incubated at 37°C in a humidified atmosphere of 95% air, 5% CO_2 for 24-48 hrs. Following 24-48 hrs of incubation period, the adherent cells were detached using Trypsin-EDTA solution 1X/0.25% (HiMedia Labs, Mumbai, India). Cell count was carried out using the Luna automated cell counter (Logos Biosystems, India) based on trypan blue dye exclusion method.

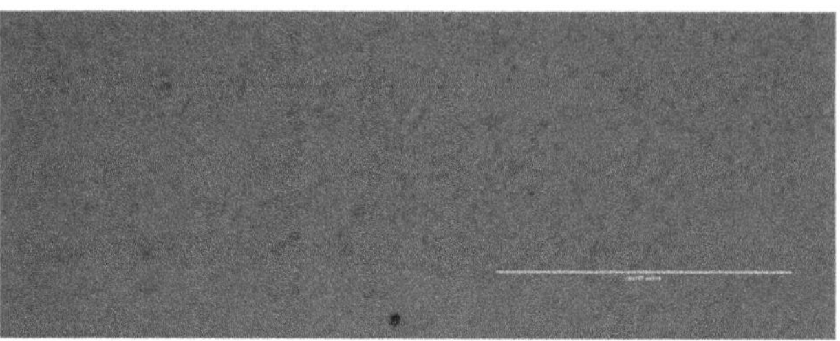

Fig 1: Image of MCF-7 cell lines

In Vitro Cell Viability Assay (MTT Assay)

Cytotoxicity of the synthesised AgNPs on the cancer cells lines was determined using MTT (3-(4,5-Dimethylthiazol-2-yl)-2,5-diphenyltetrazolium bromide) assay.

Under Normoxia conditions: (normal atmospheric oxygen conditions i.e, 21%)

The MTT [3-(4, 5-dimethylthiazol-2-yl)-2,5-diphenyl tetrazolium bromide] assay is a test that allows the measurement of cell viability/proliferation. MTT is a yellow dye that is converted to formazan/rezarin, an insoluble purple compound, by the activity of intracellular mitochondrial succinatedehydrogenase enzymes. The conversion is only able to take place in living cells therefore the amount of formazan produced is directly related to the number of viable cells present. The cells are ruptured and the formazan solubilized using a solubilization solution. The absorbance of the resultant solution is read at 570nm and cell viability was calculated as a percentage of viable cells at different test concentrations relative to the control (untreated) cells using the following formula;

$$\%\ \text{of cell viability} = \frac{A_{570}\ \text{of treated cells}}{A_{570}\ \text{of control cells}} \times 100$$

The MTT assay was performed using 200µL suspensions of each cell line which were seeded in 96-well microplates (Corning®, USA) at a density of 25,000 cells/ well and incubated for 24hrs, after which the cells were exposed to an increasing concentration of AgNPs (25, 50, 100, 125 and 150µg/mL) for 24 hrs. The AgNPs-untreated cells were used as controls for the experiment. All cells were seeded in duplicates and incubated in a CO_2 incubator (atmospheric with 5% CO_2 and 37°C temperature). 10 µl of 10% MTT dye (HiMedia Labs, Mumbai, India) was added to each well and cells incubated at 37°C with 5% CO_2, 95% air for 3 hrs. The cells were viewed under a light microscope to observe if formazan had accumulated inside the cell. The culture medium was aspirated and 100µL dimethlyl sulfoxide (DMSO; Sigma-Aldrich, India) was added to each well followed by gentle pipetting to lyse the cells. Cell viability was determined by measuring the absorbance on an ELISA microplate reader (SPECTROstar Nano, BMG LABTECH, Germany) at 570nm. Viability was calculated as a percentage of viable cells at different test concentrations relative to the control (untreated) cells (% cell viability = (A_{570} of treated cells / A_{570} of control cells) ×100%). The AgNPs concentration that resulted in 50% inhibition of cell growth was calculated as the half maximal inhibitory concentration (IC_{50}) by constructing a dose-response curve.

Under Hypoxia Conditions (Low oxygen conditions *i.e.*, 2%)

The above procedure is repeated with MCF cell lines and incubated in a CO_2 incubator at atmospheric with 5% CO_2, 2% O_2 and 37°C temperature (low oxygen conditions).

IC_{50}: Value Determination

A basic and simple method for calculation of the IC_{50} is done by linear interpolation between the concentrations just above and just beneath 50% inhibition in the dose response curve (= two flanking points). The IC_{50}: Inhibitory concentration at 50% inhibition for each cell line was determined by using the spectrophotometric results of five different AgNPs concentrations (25, 50, 100, 125 and 150µg/mL) for which a linear curve fit was generated. Cell viability percentages (y-axis) were plotted against increasing concentrations of AgNPs on the x-axis. IC_{50} value was estimated by using the linear equation

$$y = mx + c$$

Where;

y = % of inhibition
x = concentration
c = constant
m = coefficient

50 is substituted for y, yielding x as the IC_{50} value.

Reactive Oxygen Species (ROS) Measurement

The intracellular generation of ROS (superoxide) was measured using a cell permeable fluorescent marker dihydroethidium (DHE). DHE upon oxidation by superoxide anions forms a red fluorescent product (2-hydroxyethidium) within the nucleus, intercalating the DNA (Julie Nijmeh *et al.* 2010). It can be detected by fluorescent microscopy with maximum excitation and emission spectra of 518nm and 605nm respectively.

2mL cell suspension in a 6-well plate with cover slips, at a cell density of 1-2X10^5 cells per well was seeded and allowed to grow for 24h at 37°C, 5% CO_2. Silver nanoparticles was added at the concentration of 75µg/ml (1ml solution) and incubated for 24h, 37°C, 5% CO_2. Following treatment, the cells were washed 1-2 times with 1mL PBS and stained the cells with 20µM DHE (1mL per well) and incubated for 30-45 mins at 37°C, in dark. The cells were washed 1-2 times with 1mL PBS, followed by addition of 1mL PBS. Images were captured using fluorescent microscope (EVOS FL, Life Technologies, India) with appropriate channel settings.

Flow Cytometry Analysis

Flow cytometry is a technology that simultaneously measures and then analyzes multiple physical characteristics of single particles, usually cells, as they flow in a fluid stream through a beam of light.

In the flow cytometer, particles are carried to the laser intercept in a fluid stream. Any suspended particle or cell from 0.2–150 micrometers in size is suitable for analysis. Cells from solid tissue must be disaggregated before analysis. The portion of the fluid stream where particles are located is called the sample core. When particles pass through the laser intercept, they scatter laser light. Any fluorescent molecules present on the particle fluoresce. The scattered and fluorescent light is collected by appropriately positioned lenses. A combination of beam splitters and filters steers the scattered and fluorescent light to the appropriate detectors. The detectors produce electronic signals proportional to the optical signals striking them. The data are collected and stored in the computer. This data can be analyzed to provide information about subpopulations within the sample (Givan AL, 1992).

Flow Cytometric Analysis of Apoptosis and Necrosis Using Annexin V-FITC/PI Staining

Apoptosis is a normal programmed process that occurs during the life cycle of the cell. The process is characterized by specific morphologic changed such as loss of plasma membrane asymmetry that is the earliest sign of the apoptosis and this is usually used to detect apoptosis and necrosis in cells. In apoptotic cells, phospholipid phosphatidylserine (PS) in the membrane is translocated from the inner to outer plasma membrane which allows PS to bind with Annexin V which can be conjugated to a fluorochrome and detected during apoptosis observed by microscope. While the membrane of dead and damaged cells are permeable to propidium iodied (PI) consequently late apoptosis in cells and necrosis in cells are detected both Annexin V and PI. The AnnexinV-PI assay allows determination of healthy cells (annexin V-, PI-); early apoptotic cells (annexin V+, PI-) and necrotic cells (annexin V -, PI +) using the Annexin V-FITC kit (Sigma). The kit allows detection of Annexin V bound to apoptotic cells with fluorescein isothiocyante (FITC) which labels phosphatidylserine sites on the membrane surface while propidium iodide (PI) labels the DNA of necrotic cells, having permeable cell membranes.

Cells at density of 1-2X10^5 per well was seeded and cultured in a 6-well plate (Corning®, USA) for 24h at 37°C in 5% CO_2 humidified atmosphere and were later exposed to 75μg/ml AgNPs for 24h. Cells treated with 5μM 5-Fluoro Uracil (5-FU; Sigma Aldrich, India) and 200mM H_2O_2 were used as positive controls. After incubation, both attached and detached cells were harvested and washed once with 1X cold buffer and once with 1X Annexin V binding buffer (10mM HEPES, 140mM NaCl, 2.5mM $CaCl_2$, 0.1% FBS, pH 7.4). Cells were then suspended in 100μL binding buffer at 1X10^5 cells/ml concentration and stained with 5μL Annexin V-FITC. This was followed by an incubation period of 10-15 min at room temperature (RT) in dark. After incubation, the cells were washed with binding buffer and fixed with 4% PFA (Paraformaldehyde, Life Technologies, India)-0.1% Triton-X 100 (HiMedia Labs, Mumbai, India) for 10-15 min at room temperature.

After incubation the cells were washed with binding buffer and subjected to 0.25-0.5 mg/ml RNase (HiMedia Labs, Mumbai, India) treatment for 20mins at 37°C. Cells were then washed and suspended in binding buffer and stained with 5μL of 10μg/mL PI and incubated for 10-15 minutes at RT. Following incubation with PI for 10-15 minutes at RT, cells were suspended in 400μL of 1X Annexin-binding buffer and the apoptotic/necrotic populations were analysed by flow cytometer (MACSQuant Analyser, Miltenyi Biotec, Germany).

Results

Cytotoxic Studies of AgNPs

The cell density was estimated about 1-2X10^5 cells by the trypan blue dye exclusion method. Fresh cell lines at the density of 1-2X10^5 were used to each experiment.

Cell Viability

Cell viability assay is one of the vital steps in analysing the cellular response to toxic compounds, playing fundamental roles in determining the cell death and survival rates and assessing the metabolic activity. In our study, MTT assay method was applied to determine the inhibitory activity of AgNPs against the mammalian cell lines of MCF-7 under normoxia and hypoxia conditions. MTT is a yellow color dye which was reduced into purple colored formazan product by the action of mitochondrial succinate dehydrogenase enzyme.

MTT (Yellow color) — Mitochondrial Succinate dehydrogenase — Formazan (purple color)

The amount of purple colored formazan is directly related to the percentage of cell viability both under normoxia and hypoxia conditions. Normoxia is the normal atmospheric conditions, where Hypoxia literally means "low oxygen," but is defined as a deficiency in the amount of oxygen that reaches the tissues of the body. Hypoxic regions can develop as a tumour grows beyond the ability of its blood supply to deliver oxygen to the full extent of the tumour, exacerbated by vascular spasm or compression caused by increased interstitial fluid pressure. The hypoxia inducible factors (HIFs) are the key mediators of the cellular response to hypoxia. Hypoxia plays an important role in normal development and disease progression, including the growth of solid tumours.

In vitro Cytotoxicity of AgNPs in MCF-7 cells were done in dose-dependent manner ranging the concentration of AgNPs from 25 to 125μg/ml. The MTT dye was yellowish in color before incubation and turned into purple color after 24 hours of incubation. The intensity of purple color was decreased in the wells with the increased concentration of AgNPs. Decreased color intensity was the indication of increased death of cells. In other words increment of AgNPs concentration the viability decreased in all the four cell lines shown in dose-dependent curves. From the results, it is concluded that, the synthesized AgNPs were inducing Cytotoxicity in MCF-7 lines even under hypoxic conditions. This indicated that AgNPs were suggested to use in treatment of solid tumours. From the dose-dependent curves the half maximum inhibitory concentrations (IC50) values were determined. Dose-dependent Curves

Table 1: AgNPs vs MCF-7- Normoxia

OD 570nm	Untreated cells /Control	AgNPs μg/ml				
		25	50	75	100	125
1	0.956	1.002	0.968	0.637	0.559	0.212
2	0.935	0.908	0.731	0.454	0.405	0.157
Mean OD	0.9455	0.955	0.8495	0.5455	0.482	0.1845
% of viability	100	101	87.95	49.89	41.9	4.51

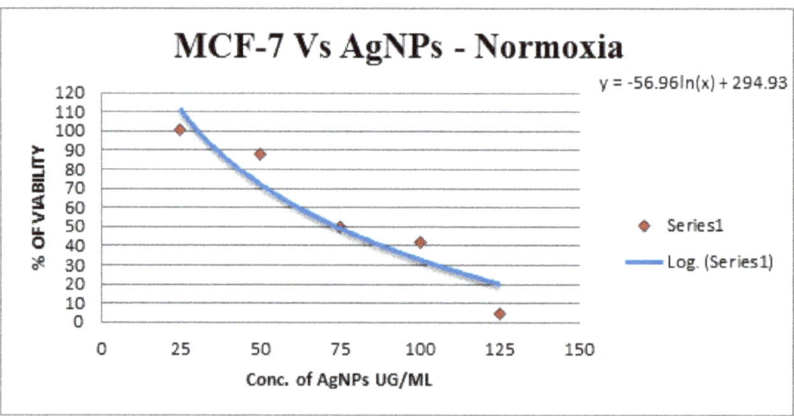

Fig 2: Dose-dependent curve of AgNPs Vs MCF-7 shows decreasing the percentage of cell viability with increasing concentration of AgNPs from 25 to 125µg/ml under normoxia.

Table 2: AgNPs Vs MCF-7- Hypoxia

OD 570nm	Untreated cells/ Control	AgNPs µg/ml				
		25	50	75	100	125
1	0.947	1.137	0.866	0.579	0.504	0.745
2	1.042	1.005	0.82	0.611	0.471	0.169
Mean OD	0.9945	1.071	0.843	0.595	0.4875	0.457
% of viability	100	108	82.76	54.45	42.12	38.69

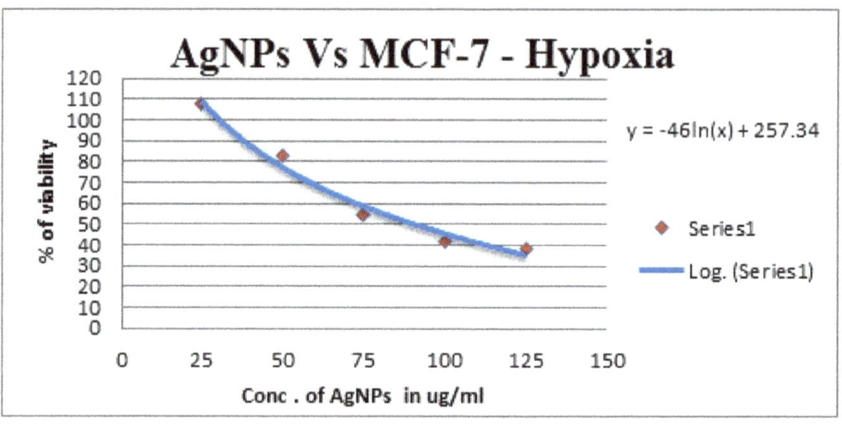

Fig 3: Dose - dependent curve of AgNPs Vs MCF-7 is showing decreasing the percentage of cell viability with increasing concentration of AgNPs from 25 to 125µg/ml under hypoxia.

Determination of IC_{50} Values

The half-maximal inhibitory concentrations (IC_{50} values) of AgNPs required to cause mortality of 50% cell population were determined by using a linear curve, where the cell viability percentages were plotted against increasing doses. IC_{50} values were calculated using the following leaner formula.

$$y = mx + c$$

Where, "y" is the half-maximal inhibitory concentration so, 50 was substituted for "y", "x" and "c" values were taken from the Excel graph and determined the "m" value which is nothing but the half-maximal inhibitory concentrations (IC_{50} values), using the following formula

$$m = \frac{y - c}{x}$$

The complete cell inhibition (99 %) of breast cancer cell lines was obtained after 48 h exposure to silver nanoparticles by dose dependent manner. The IC_{50} of cell inhibition of silver nanoparticles was observed at 82.36 μg/ml under normoxia and 96.20 μg/ml under hypoxia conditions. These results evidence the dose- and time-dependent increase in cytotoxicity. The IC_{50} value predicts that the nanosilver proves to be a promising drug for chemotherapeutic treatment even under hypoxic conditions. Shweta R *et al.* (2016) synthesized the silver nanoparticles by physical method was shown the 50% growth inhibition concentration as 178 μg/ml against the MCF-7cell lines.

Table 3: IC_{50} values of silver nanoparticles (AgNPs) in different cell lines revealed by the MTT assay-based dose-response curve.

S.No	Cancer Cell Type	IC50 values Normoxia (μg/ml)	IC50 values Hypoxia (μg/ml)
1	MCF-7	82.36	96.20

Role of AgNPs in Oxidative Stress

ROS is an oxidative stress which will cause cell injury. Generally, mitochondria are involved in the cell's response to oxidative stress. There are several steps in the path of oxygen reduction in mitochondrial electron transport chain. In the path of electron transfer some of the electrons are leak out of the system, moving from succinate to molecular oxygen to produce reactive oxygen species (ROS) and super oxide radical ($\cdot O_2^-$). The super oxide free radical thus generated $\cdot O_2^-$, is very reactive and can damage enzymes, membrane lipids and nucleic acids. To prevent oxidative damage by super oxide radical, cells have several forms of the enzyme superoxide dismutase, which catalyzes the reaction.

$$2O_2^- + 2H^+ \rightarrow H_2O_2 + O_2$$

$$H_2O_2 + 2H^+ \rightarrow 2e^- + 2H_2O$$

The hydrogen peroxide (H_2O_2) generated by this reaction is rendered harmless by the action of glutathione peroxidase (David L. Nelson and Michael M. Cox, 5th edition).

Oxidative stress is also a common mechanism of cell damage induced by nanoparticles (Xia *et al.* 2008). In the case of AgNPs, several studies have demonstrated that AgNPs have the ability to promote oxidative stress (Asharani *et al.* 2009;). Toxic agents increase the rate of superoxide anion production, either by blocking the electron transport or by accepting an electron from a respiratory carrier and transferring it to molecular oxygen without inhibiting the respiratory chain (Turrens 2003). Inhibition of respiratory chain is expected to cause decrease in

ATP synthesis. Deposition of AgNPs in mitochondria can alter normal functioning of mitochondria by disrupting the electron transport chain, ultimately resulting in ROS and low ATP yield. ROS are highly reactive and result in oxidative damage to proteins and DNA. Hence it is vital to investigate genome stability in cells with significantly higher ROS production (Asharani *et al.* 2009).

It is possible that surface oxidation of AgNP, upon contact with cell culture medium or proteins in the cytoplasm, liberates Ag ions that could amplify the toxicity. Reactions between H_2O_2 and AgNPs are presumed to be one of the factors causing Ag ions to release *in vivo*. Similar activity in cobalt and nickel nanoparticles has been reported. They release the corresponding ions that enhance toxicity (Kumar 2006).

A Possible Chemical Reaction Involves

$$2Ag + H_2O_2 + 2H+ \rightarrow Ag+ + 2H_2O \rightarrow E^0 = 0.17\ V$$

Half-reaction

$$H_2O_{2(aq)} + 2H^+ + 2e- \rightarrow H_2O_{(1)} \rightarrow E^0 = +1.77\ V$$

$$2Ag+(s) \rightarrow Ag+_{(aq)} + 2e- \quad E^0 = 2(-0.8)\ V$$

In this study, the role of AgNPs in oxidative stress was established using the ROS-specific DHE staining method. DHE (Dihydroethidium) is a cell permeable blue fluorescent marker in the reduced form, which upon oxidation by ROS yields the red-fluorescent product 2-hydroxyethidium (Julie Nijmeh *et al.* 2010). The MCF-7 cell lines treated with 200mM H_2O_2 treated cells were used as positive control. The activity of AgNPs was compared with 5-fluoro uracil (5FU), an anticancer drug which is widely used in treatment of cancer. Untreated cells which did not show fluorescence in the nucleus with DHE stain were used as standards to analyse the ROS production in treated cells. In the current investigation four cell lines were treated with 75 μg/ml of synthesized AgNPs and compared with 5FU in ROS production. The cells treated with 200mM H_2O_2, 5μM 5-FU and 75 μg/ml AgNPs showed red fluorescence in the nucleus.

From the Fig. 3 untreated cell was showing negligible amount of red fluorescent due to cell damage while handling or any other cause. Silver nanoparticle treated cells were showing almost more or equal fluorescent dye with that of 5FU. Thus, ROS production by AgNPs was maximum when compared with 5FU. There is a significant increase in the levels of ROS was observed in comparison to the H_2O_2 treated controls. From the results it can be analyzed that, the synthesized silver nanoparticles was successfully inducing reactive oxygen stress in the cancerous cell lines and stopping the cell proliferation. Our results were supported by many other scientists; Brown *et al.* (2004) analyzed the importance of ROS in triggering many cellular pathways which can lead to cellular death, including cytokine activation and caspase activation (Kim *et al.* 2009). They can also cause damage to the nuclear DNA by altering the chemical structure of the nucleotide bases and the deoxyribosyl backbone (Cooke *et al.* 2003). As a result, intracellular ROS generation upon AgNPs exposure is a significant factor to its cytotoxicity.

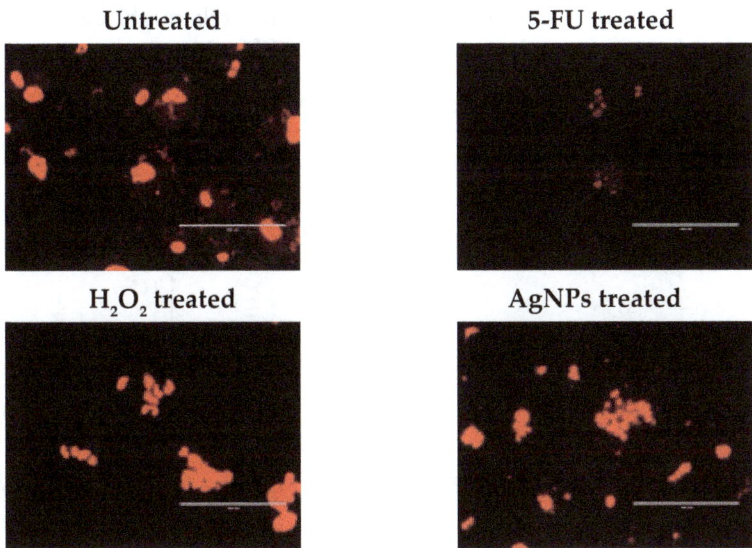

Fig 4: a) MCF-7 cell were treated with 5 μM 5FU, 200mM H_2O_2 and M75μg/ml AgNP for 24 hours and the expression of oxygen free radicals was analyzed by labeling with 20μM dihydroethidium (DHE).

Analysis of Apoptosis/Necrosis using Flow Cytometry

Annexin V-FITC/PI Apoptosis/Necrosis Assay

ROS generation could cause cell death by two distinct mechanisms, either apoptosis or necrosis. The ability of silver nanoparticles to induce apoptosis (programmed cell death) was assessed using Annexin V-FITC/PI staining. This assay is used to determine membrane integrity based on phosphatidylserine migration to the extracellular surface of apoptotic cells when disruption occurs.

In our study, the AgNPs ability to induce toxicity was evaluated using the Annexin V-FITC/PI double staining method with the flow cytometer, which revealed the extent and mode of cell death. 5FU treated cells were used as positive control and untreated cells was used as standards. A statistical analysis was made using the MACSQuant software and a dot plot, the respective quadrants describes:

(1) Percentages of viable cells (AV−/PI−; LL1),

(2) Early apoptotic cells (AV+/PI−; LR1),

(3) Late apoptotic and necrotic cells (AV+/PI+; UR1) and

(4) Residual damaged cells (AV−/PI+; UL1).

The data indicated that the exposure of cells to AgNPs could lead to apoptosis, in particular early apoptosis.

From the flow cytometric studies MCF-7 cells were showing 99.6% of apoptosis, 0.02% of late apoptosis and there was no residual damage when treated with AgNPs. MCF-7 cells treated with 5FU were showing 99.4% of apoptosis, 0.48% of late apoptosis and there0.16% of residual damage Compared with 5FU; synthesized silver nanoparticles were showing 0.02% more apoptosis in MCF-7 cells. Untreated cells were also showing 0.03% of apoptosis, 0.3% of late apoptosis and 11.3% of residual damage. It was due to the cells might be damaged during process and might be stained with Annexin-V/PI stain.

MCF-7 (Human Breast Cancer Cell Line) -ANNEXIN-V vs PI

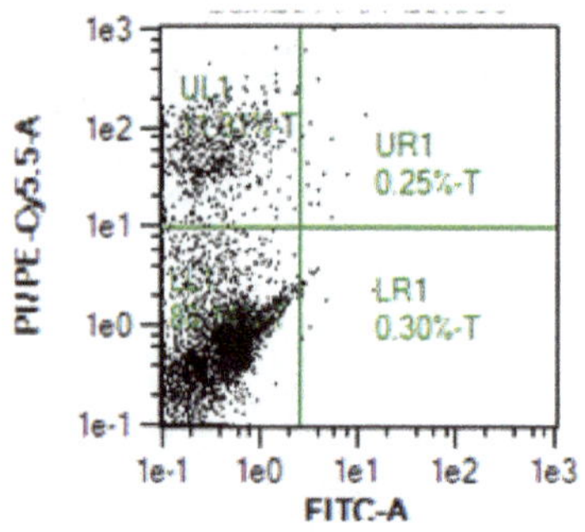

a). Control: ANNEXIN V-FITC/PI

LL1 = 88.1%; UL1 = 11.3; UR1 = 0.3%; LR1= 0.3%

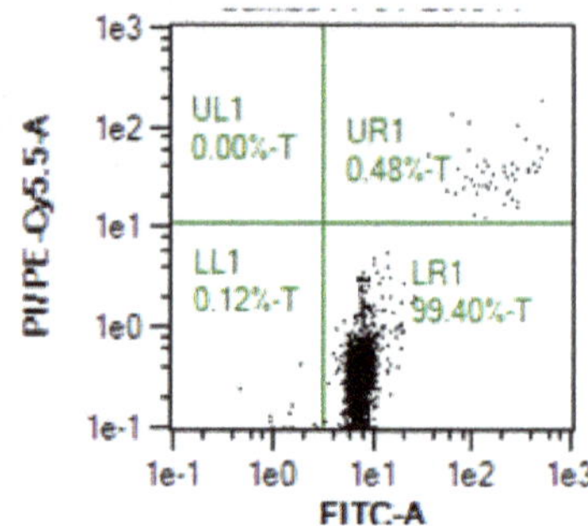

b). 5FU: ANNEXIN V- FITC/PI

LL1 = 0.12%; UL1 = 0.16; UR1 = 0.48%; LR1= 99.40%

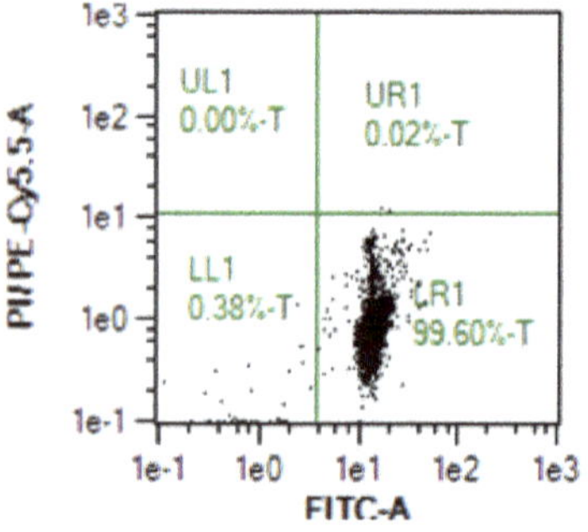

c). AgNPs: ANNEXIN- V- FITC/PI

LL1 = 0.4%; UL1 = 0.00%; UR1 = 0.02%; LR1= 99.60%

Fig 5: MCF-7 cells were untreated a), and treated with 5μM 5FU for 24 hours b), 75μg/ml AgNP for 24 hours c). Cells were then labelled with Annexin V-FITC and 5ug/ml of PI. Statistical data were extracted from the dot plots using MACS Quant software, based on the percentages of viable (AV−/PI−; LL1), early apoptotic (AV+/PI−; LR1), apoptotic (AV+/PI+; UR1) and residual damaged (AV−/PI+; UL1) cells are shown in the respective quadrants.

Table 4: Statistical data of early apoptosis, late apoptosis and residual damage in MCF-7 cell lines after 24 hours treatment with 5FU and AgNPs respectively with standard /control.

% of MCF-7 cells				
	Live -LL1	**Early apoptotic-LR1**	**Late apoptotic/Necrotic -UR1**	**Residual damage – UL1**
Control	88.1	0.3	0.3	11.3
5-FU	0.12	99.4	0.48	0.16
AgNPs	0.4	99.6	0.02	0

Conclusion

Investigations from the current research, silver nanoparticles synthesized from *C. glutamicum* ATCC 13032, showing elevated apoptotic cell population in the tested cancerous cell lines. The synthesized AgNPs were exbiting 99.6% in MCF cells. Compared with 5FU, AgNPs were extreamly effective to cause apoptotic cell death.

The overall results indicated that the biologically synthesized AgNPs have antiproliferative activity through induction of apoptosis in MCF cancerous cell lines, suggesting that biologically synthesized AgNPs might be a potential alternative agent for cancer therapy. This study demonstrates the possibility of using AgNPs to inhibit the growth of the tumour cells and their cytotoxicity for potential therapeutic treatments and offers a new method to develop molecule for cancer therapy. Finally, cost effectiveness, biocompatibility, and facileness to modify these silver nanoparticles make them viable choice in future biomedical applications.

Hence, the data represented in our study contribute to a novel and unexplored area of nanomaterials as alternative medicine in the treatment of solid cancer.

References

Asharani PV, Low Kah Mun G, Hande MP, Valiyaveettil S. (2009). Cytotoxicity and genotoxicity of silver nanoparticles in human cells. *ACS Nano*. 24: 279-90.

Bilberg, K., Døving, K.B., Beedholm, K., Baatrup, E. (2011). Silver nanoparticles disrupt olfaction in Crucian carp (*Carassius carassius*) and Eurasian perch (*Perca fluviatilis*). *Aquat. Toxicol*. 104:145–152.

Brown DM, Donaldson K, Borm PJ, Schins RP, Dehnhard M, Gilmour P, Jimenez LA, Stone V. (2004). Calcium and ROS-mediated activation of transcription factors and TNF- a cytokine gene expression in macrophages exposed to ultrafine particles. *Am. J. Physiol. Lung Cell. Mol. Physiol*. 286: 344– 353.

Castranova, V. (2011). Overview of current toxicological knowledge of engineered nanoparticles. *J. Occup. Environ. Med*. 53: S14–S17.

Cooke MC, Evans MD, Dizdaroglu M, Lunec J. (2003). Oxidative DNA damage: mechanisms, mutation, and disease. *FASEB Journal*. 17: 1195–1214.

David L. Nelson and Michael M. Cox. (2008) Lehninger Principles of biochemistry. 5th Ed., W.H.Freeman & Co Ltd, pp. 715.

Givan AL (1992), Flow Cytometry: First Principles. 1st Ed., New York, NY: Wiley-Liss; (ISBN 978-0-471-38224-9), pp.202.

Gowramma B, Avadhani G.S, Rafi M., Chamundeswaramma K.V., Muralidhara Rao D. (2014). Production and scrutiny of silver nanoparticles from Corynebacterium glutamicum ATCC13032 and antimicrobial sensitivity assessment. *Asian J of Biological and Life sciences*. 3:81-89.

Julie Nijmeh, Aigul Moldobaeva, and Elizabeth M. Wagner (2010). Role of ROS in ischemia-induced lung angiogenesis. *Am J Physiol Lung Cell Mol Physiol*. 299:535–541.

Kathiravan V, Ravi S, Ashokkumar S. (2014). Synthesis of silver nanoparticles from Melia dubia leaf extract and their in vitro anticancer activity. *Spectrochim Acta Part A: Mol Biomol Spectrosc*. 130:116–121. doi: 10.1016/j.saa.2014.03.107.

Kim S, Choi JE, Choi J, Chung KH, Park K, Yi J, Ryu DY. (2009), Oxidative stress-dependent toxicity of silver nanoparticles in human hepatoma cells. *Toxicol In Vitro* 23: 1076-1084.

Kumar C. (2006). Nanomaterials-Toxicity, Health and Environmental Issues; Vol. 5. Wiley- VCH Verlag GmbH & Co: Weinheim, Germany,

Lokina S, Stephen A, Kaviyarasan V, Arulvasu C, Narayanan V. (2014). Cytotoxicity and antimicrobial activities of green synthesized silver nanoparticles. *Eur J Med Chem*. 76:256–263. doi: 10.1016/j.ejmech.2014.02.010.

Nagajyothi PC, Sreekanth TVM, Lee JI, Lee KD. (2014) Mycosynthesis: antibacterial, antioxidant and antiproliferative activities of silver nanoparticles synthesized from *Inonotus obliquus* (*Chaga mushroom*) extract. *J Photochem Photobiol B Biol*. 130:299–304. doi: 10.1016/j.jphotobiol.2013.11.022.

Ranjitham AM, Suja R, Caroling G, Tiwari S. (2013). *In vitro* evaluation of antioxidant, antimicrobial, anticancer activities and characterisation of *Brassica oleracea*. var. *bortrytis*. L. synthesized silver nanoparticles. *Int J Pharm Pharm Sci*. 5:239–251.

Reddy NJ, Nagoor Vali D, Rani M, Rani SS. Evaluation of antioxidant, antibacterial and cytotoxic effects of green synthesized silver nanoparticles by Piper longum fruit. *Mater Sci Eng* C.;34(1):115–122. doi: 10.1016/j.msec.2013.08.039.

Shweta R, Rajnish K, Rajukumar K, Shreyas P. (2016). Sonali Saha and Qureshi M.S,.Study of anti-cancer properties of green silver nanoparticles against MCF-7 breast cancer cell lines, progress in Biomaterials. 5:03-14 DOI: https://doi.org/10.1515/gps-2015-0104.

Sriram MI, Kalishwaralal K, Barathmanikanth S, Gurunathani S. (2012.) Size-based cytotoxicity of silver nanoparticles in bovine retinal endothelial cells. *Nanosci Methods*. 1:56–77. doi: 10.1080/17458080.2010.547878.

Turrens JF. (2003). Mitochondrial Formation of Reactive Oxygen Species. *J. Physiol.* 552: 335–344.

Wang B, Yang Q, Wang Y, Li Z. (2014). The toolbox of designing nanoparticles for tumors. *Mini Rev Med Chem*. 14:707–716. doi: 10.2174/1389557514666140820122307.

Wang B, Yang Q, Wang Y, Li Z. (2014). The toolbox of designing nanoparticles for tumors. *Mini Rev Med Chem*. 14:707–716. doi: 10.2174/1389557514666140820122307.

Xi Feng Z, Wei S, Sangiliyandi G. (2016). Silver nanoparticles-mediated cellular responses in various cell lines: an *in vitro* model. *Int J Mol Sci*. 17:1603–1629.

Xia T, Kovochich M, Liong M. (2008). Comparsion of the mechanism of toxicity of zinc oxide and cerium oxide nanoparticles based on dissolution and oxidative stress properties. *ACS Nano*. 2:2121–34.

Innovations in Biochemical Techniques (2020) : Page no. 65-70
ASTRAL INTERNATIONAL (P) LTD., New Delhi - 110002

Chapter 5

Efficient Synthesis and Antimicrobial Studies of 2-oxo-2*H*-Selenopyrano [2,3-*b*] Quinoline-3-Carbonitriles

B. P. Nandeshwarappa[a], S. O. Sadashiv[b], Sharangouda J. Patil[c] and G. K. Prakash[d]

Department of PG Studies and Research in Chemistry, Shivagangothri, Davangere University, Davanagere, Karnataka - 577 007 [a], Department of PG Studies and Research in Food Technology, Shivagangothri, Davangere University, Davanagere, Karnataka - 577 007, India. [b] Department of Life Sciences, School of Sciences, Garden City University, Bengaluru - 560 049, India. [c] Department of Chemistry, Bapuji Institute of Engineering and Technology Davanagere - 560 004, India [d]
Email: belakatte@gmail.com.

Abstract

Substituted 2-oxo-2H-selenopyrano [2,3-*b*] quinoline-3-carbonitriles 4a-e were synthesised by the treatment of 3-formyl-2-selenoquinolines 3a-e with ethyl cyanoacetate in presence of piperidine. The newly synthesised compounds were characterized by elemental analysis, IR, ^{1}H NMR and mass spectral data. The synthesized compounds 4a-e were evaluated for antimicrobial activities. Among the compounds tested, 4d and 4e were highly active against *S. aureus* and *M. roseus*.

Keywords: *Antimicrobial activities, ethyl cyanoacetate, 3-formyl-2-chloroquinoline, 3-formyl-2-selenoquinoline, Selenopyrano[2,3-b]quinoline and pharmaceutical applications.*

Introduction

Selenium is an element, which resembles the sulfur in terms of its chemical properties. It has been successfully introduced into organic compounds either as an electrophile or as a nucleophile. Humans and animals need selenium for various biological functions, which involve some organoselenium compounds (Rayman, 2000). It is also known that many selenium containing organic molecules are antibacterial and antifungal agents. Organoselenium compounds have been known for a long time as versatile reagents in organic chemistry. Sulfur and selenium are considered to be isosteric as defined by Langmuir (1919), Erlenmeyer, (1948). Even though sulfur and selenium are considered to be isosteric, reports about selenium containing hetrocycles are relatively scares (Nandha Kumar *et al.*, 2003, Lalezari *et al.*, 1974, Singh, 1992).

In recent years, many exciting research results have indicated that selenium has gained the attention of scientists working in a variety of fields. The interest in selenium-containing compounds has increased not only because of their reactivites and chemical properties (Sommen *et al.*, 2005, Klayman, 1973, Paulmier, 1986, Renson *et al.*, 1986, Litvinov, 1997), but also because of their pharmaceutical applications (Passwaters, 1980, Wendel, 1989, Burk, 1994).

During the past few decades, interest has been rapidly growing in gaining insight into the properties and transformations of these heterocycles. It is evident from literature that, substituted quinolines are important and widely used heterocyclic compounds in heterocyclic chemistry.

In continuation of our research program directed towards the studies on selenium compounds (Kiran *et al.*, 2006) and other heterocycles. (Nandeshwarappa *et al.*, 2006 a,b,c, 2005, 2007, Nandeshwarappa, 2017 a,b,c,d,e,f, Nandeshwarappa and Manjunatha Swamy, 2017) Their wide range of biological properties led promoted us to investigate the synthesis and antimicrobial activities of selenopyrano[2,3-b] quinolines.

Results and Discussions

In this contribution, we focused our attention on the synthesis of 2-oxo-2H-selenopyrano[2,3-*b*]quinoline-3-carbonitrile. At first the key intermediates 3-formyl-2-chloroquinoline (Meth-Kohn *et al.*, 1981) and 3-formyl-2-selenoquinolines (Prakash Naik *et al.*, 2007) have been prepared from available reported methods. Synthetic strategy involving the condensation the 3-formyl-2-seleno quinoline with ethyl cyanoacetate 3c in presence of catalytic amount of piperidine.

The ^{1}H NMR spectrum of 4a revealed a multiplet at δ 8.6-9.7 ppm due to six aromatic protons. The IR spectrum of 4a exhibited absorption bands at 1620 cm^{-1} corresponding to newly formed selenopyrano carbonyl group and 2222 cm^{-1} corresponding to cyano group attached to selenopyrano ring.

Experimental

IR spectra were taken on a Perkin Elmer 157 Infrared spectrophotometer. The 1H NMR spectra (300 MHz) were recorded on a Bruker supercon FT NMR instrument using TMS as internal standard and mass spectra on a Jeol JMS-D 300 Mass spectrometer operating at 70 eV. Melting points were determined in open capillary and are uncorrected. Purity of the compounds was checked by TLC on silica gel and were purified by column chromatography.

Synthesis of 2-oxo-2H-selenopyrano[2,3-*b*]quinoline-3-carbonitriles (4a-e)

A mixture of 3-formyl-2-seleno quinoline29 3a (0.01 mole) and ethyl cyanoacetate, (0.01 mole) containing piperidine (5 drops) were taken in around bottomed flask containing 100ml of acetonitrile. The contents of the reaction mixture were refluxed over 3 hours. The completion of reaction was monitored by means of TLC; the reaction mixture was poured into crushed ice, stirred well, filtered and the crude product 4a was either recrystallized from ethyl acetate/

chloroform or subjected to silica gel chromatography using ethyl acetate/carbon tetrachloride, 8:2 as the eluent.

4a. 2-oxo-2H-selenopyrano[2,3-b]quinoline-3-carbonitrile

Solid, Yield 79%. mp. 232◦C; ^{1}H NMR (300 MHz, DMSO-d6) δ (ppm): 8.67-9.77 (m, 6H, Ar-H); IR (KBr) ν (cm−1): 1620 (C=O), 2222 (CN); [M+], 285. Calcd. (%) for C14H6N2OSe: C; 54.75. H; 2.12, N; 9.29, Found: C; 54.85. H; 2.16, N; 9.21.

4b.7-Methoxy-2-oxo-2H-selenopyrano[2,3-b]quinoline-3-carbonitrile

Solid, Yield 76%. mp. 228◦C; ^{1}H NMR (300 MHz, DMSO-d6) δ (ppm): 4.20-4.31 (s, 3H, -OCH3), 7.56-8.67 (m, 5H, Ar-H); IR (KBr) ν (cm−1): 1622 (C=O), 2223 (CN); [M+], 315. Calcd. (%) for C14H8N2O2Se: C; 53.35. H; 2.56, N; 8.89, Found: C; 53.39. H; 2.61, N; 8.93.

4c. 7-Bromo-2-oxo-2H-selenopyrano[2,3-b]quinoline-3-carbonitrile

Solid, Yield 81%. mp. 238◦C; ^{1}H NMR (300 MHz, DMSO-d6) δ (ppm): 7.58-7.89 (m, 5H, Ar-H); IR (KBr) ν (cm−1): 1625 (C=O), 2221(CN); [M+], 364. Calcd. (%) for C13H5 BrN2OSe: C; 42.89, H; 1.38, N; 7.69, Found: C; 42.93, H; 1.42, N; 7.75.

4d. 7-Chloro-2-oxo-2H-selenopyrano[2,3-b]quinoline-3-carbonitrile

Solid, Yield 72%. mp. 245◦C; ^{1}H NMR (300 MHz, DMSO-d6) δ (ppm): 7.57-8.71 (m, 5H, Ar-H); IR (KBr) ν (cm−1): 1625 (C=O), 2223(CN); [M+], 319. Calcd. (%) for C13H5ClN2OSe : C; 48.85, H; 1.58, N; 8.77, Found: C; 48.89, H; 1.63, N; 8.82.

4e. 7-Nitro-2-oxo-2H-selenopyrano[2,3-b]quinoline-3-carbonitrile

Solid, Yield 71%. mp. 239◦C; ^{1}H NMR (300 MHz, DMSO-d6) δ (ppm): 7.57-8.71 (m, 5H, Ar-H); IR (KBr) ν (cm−1): 1622 (C=O), 2222(CN); [M+], 330. Calcd. (%) for C13H5N3O3Se: C; 47.29, H; 1.53, N; 12.73, Found: C; 47.33, H; 1.59, N; 12.79.

Antmicrobial Activity

The in vitro antimicrobial activity was carried out against 24 h old cultures of three bacteria by disk diffusion method (Finegold, 1982) using ampicillin as the reference. Compounds 4a-e were tested against Gram positive bacteria (Staphylococcus aureus, Micrococcus roseus), a Gram negative bacteria (Escherichia coli). The compounds were tested at a concentration of 0.001mol / ml in DMF against all organisms. The zone of inhibition was compared with the standard drug after 24 h of incubation at 25°C and measured in mm. Results are reported in Table 1, it was found that compounds 4d and 4e were highly active against *S. aureus* and *M. roseus* (gram positive) and moderately active against E. coli (gram negative), compound 4c was slightly active against M. roseus and E. coli. Compound 4e was slightly active against S. aureus and M. roseus and compounds 4a and 4b were slightly active against M. roseus. Other compounds were all inactive against these three pathogenic microorganisms. Hence further studies in these compounds are planed to obtain clinically useful agents.

Antimicrobial activity tests of 2-oxo-2H-selenopyrano[2,3-b]quinoline-3-carbonitrile (4a-e)

Comp. No	Microorganism		
	S. aureus	M. roseus	E. coli
Ampicillin	20	22	22
4a	6	8	6
4b	5	5	5
4c	3	6	5
4d	14	17	12
4e	13	14	9

Zone of inhibition was expressed in mm

Highly active +++ (inhibition zone>12 mm); Moderately active ++ (inhibition zone 9-12 mm); Slightly active + (inhibition zone 6-9 mm); Inactive - inhibition zone<6 mm).

Reaction Scheme

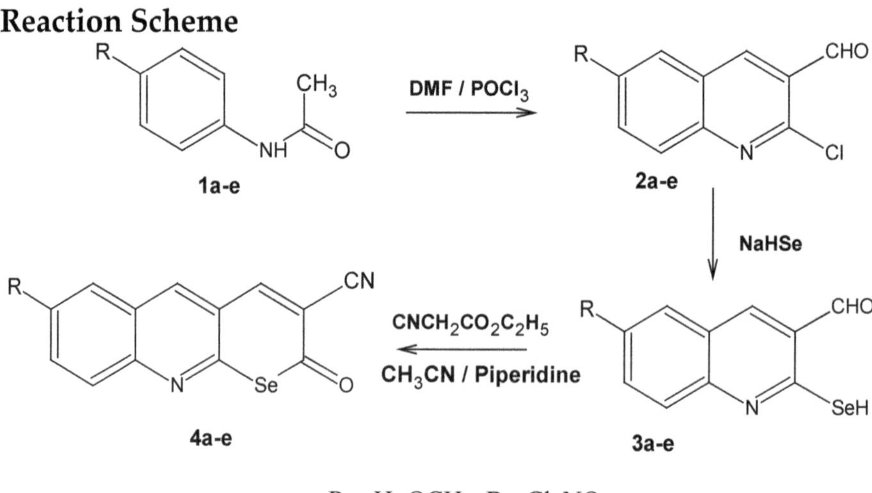

R = H, OCH_3, Br, Cl, NO_2

Fig 1: Scheme - 2-oxo-2H-selenopyrano [2,3-b] quinoline-3-carbonitriles

References

Burk, R. F., (1994). Selenium in biology and human health, Springer, New York, 181.

Erlenmeyer, H. (1948), The enlarged concept of isosterism, Bull. So. Chem. Bio., 1948, 30, 792.

Finegold, S. M., Martin, W. J., (1982), Mosby Diagnostic Microbiology,: London, 6th ed.; 450.

J. of Chem. and Chemical Scienc., 7(3), 222.

Kiran B. M., Nandeshwarappa B. P., Prakash G. K., Vaidya V. P. and Mahadevan K. M., (2007), Synthesis of new seleno substituted quinolines, *Phosphorus Sulfur and Silicon Related Elements*, 182, 993.

Kiran B. M., Nandeshwarappa B. P., Vaidya V. P. and Mahadevan K. M., (2007),Chemistry of substituted Thieno and Thiopyrano[2,3-b]quinolines. *Phosphorus Sulfur and Silicon Related Elements*, 182, 969.

Klayman D. L., Gunther W. H. H., (1973),Inorganic selenium compounds: Their chemistry and biology, 579, 629. *John Wiley & Sons, New York.*

Lalezari A., Shafiee S., and Yazdani, (1974), Selenium heterocycles. X. synthesis and antibacterial activity of pyridyl-1,2,3- thiadiazoles and pyridyl-1,2,3-selenadiazoles, *J. Pharm Sci.*, 63, 628.

Langmiur, (1919), Isomorphism, isosterism and covalence, *J. Am. Chem. Soc.*, 4, 1543.

Litvinov V. P., Dyachenko V. D., (1997), Selenium containing heterocycles, Russ. Chem. Rev., 66, 923.

Meth-Kohn O., Narin B., Tarnowski B., Hayes R., Keyzad A., Rhousati S., and Robinson A., (1981), A versatile new synthesis of quinolines and related fused pyridines. Part 9. Synthetic application of the 2-chloroquinoline-3-carbaldehydes, *J. Chem. Soc. Perkin Trans.*, 1, 2509.

Nandeshwarappa B. P. and Manjunatha Swamy H. M., (2017), New and efficient synthesis of [(3-formylquinolin-2-yl)thio]acetic acids, *J. of Chem. and Chemical Scienc*, 7(2), 131.

Nandeshwarappa B. P., (2017), An Efficient Synthesis of ethyl {[3-(hydroxymethyl) quinolin-2-yl]thio}acetate, *J. of Chem. and Chemical Scienc.*, 7(3), 242.

Nandeshwarappa B. P., (2017), Facile Synthesis of Sulfur Containing Condensed Quinolines,

Nandeshwarappa B. P., (2017), Novel Approach Towards Synthesis of Ethyl [(3-formylquinolin-2-yl) thio] acetate *J. of Chem. and Chemical Scienc.*, 7(3), 237.

Nandeshwarappa B. P., (2017), Novel Synthesis of New Thieno [2,3-b]quinoline-2-carboxylates *J. of Chem. and Chemical Scienc.*, 7(3), 230.

Nandeshwarappa B. P., (2017), Solvent free, Inorganic solid supported synthesis of Furoquinolines under Microwave irradiation: *J. of Chem. and Chemical Scienc.*, 7(1), 15.

Nandeshwarappa B. P., (2017), Synthesis of {[3-(hydroxymethyl)quinolin-2-yl] thio}acetic acid J. *of Chem. and Chemical Scienc.*, 7(3), 247.

Nandeshwarappa B. P., Arun Kumar D. B., Bhojya Naik H. S. and Mahadevan K. M., (2005), An Efficient microwave-assisted synthesis of thieno [2,3-b] quinolines under solvent-free condition, *J. Sulfur. Chem.*, 26(4-5), 373.

Nandeshwarappa B. P., Arun Kumar D. B., Kumaraswamy M. N., Ravikumar Y. S., Bhojya Naik H. S. and Mahadevan K. M., (2006), Microwave assisted synthesis of some novel thiopyrano [2,3-b] quinolines as a new class of antimicrobial agent, *Phosporous, Sulfur and Silicon*, 181, 1545.

Nandeshwarappa B. P., Aruna Kumar D. B., Bhojya Naik H. S. and Mahadevan K. M., (2006), A fast and large-scale synthesis of 3-formyl-2-mercapto quinolines, *Phosphorus Sulfur and Silicon Relat. Elem.*, 181, 1997.

Nandeshwarappa B. P., Aruna Kumar D. B., Kumaraswamy M. N., Ravi Kumar Y. S., Bhojya Naik H. S., Mahadevan K. M., (2006), Microwave assisted one pot synthesis of 8-methyl-3,6,9-triphenyl-5,6-dihydro- 9H-pyrazolo [3,4-e] [1,2,4] triazolo [3,4-b] [1,3,4] thiadiazepine, *Phosphorus Sulfur and Silicon Relat. Elem.*, 81, 1545.

Nandha Kumar R., Thamarai Selvi S, Suresh T, and Mohan P. S. (2003), Reactions of heterocyclic quinone methides: A facile entry to synthesize the alkaloid, flindersine and its analogues, *Ind. J. Chem.*, 42B, 187.

Passwaters, R. A., (1980), Selenium as food & medicine, Pivot Original Press, New Canaan.

Paulmier C., (1986), Selenium reagent and intermediates in organic synthesis, 70, Pergamon Press, Oxford.

Prakash Naik H. R., Bhojya Naik H. S., Aravinda T., Ravikumar Naik T. R., and Lamani D. S., (2007), A facile one pot synthesis of 4-methylthieno[2,3-b] quinolin-3(2H)-one and 4-methylseleno[2,3-b]quinolin-3(2H)-ones by microwave irradiation under solvent free condition. *Organic Chem., An Indian Jour.*, 3(4), 188.

Rayman, M. P. (2000), The importance of selenium to human health., Brit. Med. J. 356, 233.

Renson M., Patai Ed., Rappoport Z. (1986), The chemistry of organic selenium and tellurium compounds, 1, 339. John Wiley & Sons, New York.

Sharma K. S., Singh. S. P., (1992), Condensed heterocycles, Ind. J. Chem., 31B, 396.

Sommen G. L., Linden A., and Heimgartner H., (2005) Selenium-containing heterocycles from isoselenocyanates: cycloaddition of carbodiimides to selenazetidines, Helv. Chim. Acta., 88, 766.

Wendel, A. (1989), Selenium in biology and medicine, ed. Springer-Verlag, Berlin, 73, 318.

Innovations in Biochemical Techniques (2020) : Page no. 71-80
ASTRAL INTERNATIONAL (P) LTD., New Delhi - 110002

Chapter 6

Seismological Studies of Surface Latent Heat Flux as an Earthquake Precursor

Jeevan Kumar C M[1], Suryanshu Choudhary[1] and Shivamurthaiah M.[3]

Research scholar[1], RNT University[2], Bhopal, MP Professors, RNT University [3], Bhopal, MP Email: [1]jeevankumarcm@gmail.com, [2] csuryansh@gmail.com Contact: [1] +91 9535215335, [2] +91 9977678759.

Abstract

The association between varieties in surface inactive warmth transition (SLHF) and ocean seismic action has been an in vogue issue of later seismological investigations. Up until this point, there are two issues, how to distinguish the unusual SLHF varieties from troublesome foundation signs, and how to guarantee that the inconsistency result from seismic action. In this paper, we proposed four movable parameters for ID, arranged the association and dissect SLHF changes a while before six ocean seismic movement by utilizing every day SLHF information. Plus, we additionally quantitatively assess the long haul association between seismic movement and SLHF peculiarities for the six investigation territories over a 20 yr period going before each seismic action. The outcomes propose: (1) preceding the South Sandwich Islands, Papua, Samoa and Haiti seismic action, the SLHF varieties over their individual foundation levels have generally low amplitudes and are hard to be considered as preliminary abnormalities; (2) in the wake of evacuating the bunching impact, the greater part of the oddities before these six seismic movement are not transiently identified with any seismic action in each investigation zone in time grouping; (3) for each case, aside from Haiti, more than halfway of concentrated seismic action which were sensible notwithstanding obliterating seismic action (Mw = 5.3) had no prior varieties in SLHF; and (4) the relationship among SLHF and seismic action depends to a great extent on data rightness and parameter settings. Before any utilization of SLHF information on seismic action expectation, we recommend that oddity recognizing measures ought to be set up dependent on long haul provincial examination to wipe out is suavity. Besides, different elements which may result in SLHF varieties additionally ought to be cautiously considered.

Introduction

Among a substantial number of purported seismic movement antecedents, (for example, geomagnetism, gas arrangement and electromagnetic radiation), warm varieties have been exceptionally compelling over the most recent quite a few years. In the prior 1980s, temperature information acquired from ground meteorological stations was utilized to contemplate the association between earth-tremors and soil or air temperature changes at various profundities and rises (Hao *et al.*, 1982; Wang and Zhu, 1984). As of late, the advancement of satellite and sensor advances has permitted perception at a lot higher spatial and fleeting goals. By utilizing NOAA-AVHRR satellite warm pictures, Tronin utilized warm remote detecting information to watch unusual infrared radiation in a seismically dynamic district in focal Asia (Tronin, 1996). Practically equivalent to remotely detected pictures were likewise utilized in Russia, China, India, Mexico and different nations. Besides, warm remote detecting items have additionally been utilized in the investigation of the association between warm varieties and seismic action, for example, active long wave radiation (OLR) and temperature of dark body (TBB) (Ouzounov *et al.*, 2007; Zhang *et al.*, 2010). As a key segment of Earth's vitality spending plan, SLHF (surface dormant warmth motion) which speaks to the warmth motion coming about because of changes in water stage, has been as of late proposed as a conceivable antecedent to ocean/beach front seismic movement. Dey and Singh right off the bat found that some atypical SLHF crests a couple of days before five seismic movement that happened close to the sea, making them propose SLHF as an antecedent to seismic action in waterfront areas (Dey and Singh, 2003). In view of their disclosure, albeit a few information mining innovations, including wavelet change and spatial/fleeting congruity examination, have been subsequently acquainted with investigate the transient and spatial varieties of SLHF when seismic movement (Cervone *et al.*, 2004, 2005; Singh *et al.*, 2007), there are many of researchers as yet concentrating on point and momentary investigation. The majority of the present investigation of association between seismic movement and SLHF forerunners by and large comprises of concentrating on at least one explicit seismic action; looking at their individual day by day SLHF for a while before the seismic action to foundation esteems (determined distinctively by various creators); announcing irregularities; showing a few pictures of the variety in SLHF preceding and following the earth-tremor; and examining the spatial examples of SLHF varieties in a specific territory.

In this investigation, the assessment methodology was done in three stages: recognizing transient peculiarities dependent on different examinations; deciding whether they are seismic movement prompted inconsistencies utilizing long haul information; change a few parameters to dissect their impact on the relationship establishment. Therefore, this paper is sorted out as pursues: seismic action and SLHF items are presented in Sect. 2; the quantitative short and long haul associations are delineated, arranged and assessed in Sect. 3; the dialog is stretched out to SLHF information and related parameters to address the significance of information pertinence and limit settings in Sect. 4; and end are given in Sect 5.

Data

Seismic Events

Amid the previous decade, many appalling seismic movement happened in nearness to a sea or underneath the ocean bottom. In this paper, we think about six seismic movements: Sumatra, Papua, Samoa, Haiti, Tohoku and one east of the South Sandwich Islands (from now on alluded to as ESSI). The primary choice criteria incorporate a greatness of Mw = 7.0 or bigger, comparative central profundity in the hull and close or underneath a sea. Figure 1 demonstrates the epicentral areas of the chose seismic movement, and Table 1 gives their essential data (http://seismic activity.usgs.gov/).

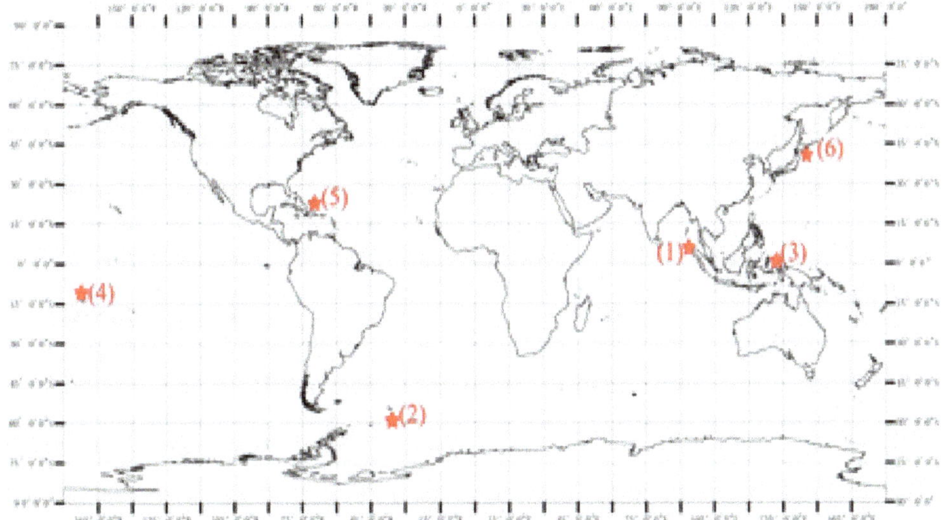

Fig 1: Areas of concentrated seismic action Index distinguishes the comparing seismic action depicted in Table 1.

Table 1: Different Concentrated Seismic Events.

Name	Time (UTC)	Location (Lon, Lat)	Magnitude (Mw)	Depth (km)	NCEP (Lon, Lat)
Sumatra	26 Dec 2004 00:58	95.92◦E, 3.295◦ N	9.0	30	51, 49
ESSI	2 Jan 2006 06:10	21.60◦W,60.957◦S	7.4	13	107, 15
Papua	3 Jan 2009 19:43	132.885◦E,0.414◦ S	7.7	17	70, 47
Samoa	29 Sep 2009 17:48	172.09◦W,15.489◦S	8.1	18	187, 39
Haiti	12 Jan 2010 21:53	72.57◦W,18.443◦N	7.0	13	134, 57
Tohoku	11mar 2011 05:46	142.36◦E,38.322◦N	9.0	32	76, 67

SLHF

Earth's surface not just retains and discharges heat by electromagnetic radiation yet additionally trades vitality with the environment through reasonable and inert warmth ex-change. The previous is brought about via air choppiness or convection, and the last is for the most part brought about by water stage changes. The expression "surface inactive warmth transition" (SLHF) is utilized to portray the motion of warmth from the outside of the land or sea to the environment that is related with the hardening, liquefying and transpiration of water (Bourras, 2006; Schulz *et al.*, 1997). Because of the homogeneity of sea medium, SLHF can be effectively used to screen heat varieties at the sea environment interface. SLHF information can be gotten in different ways. Customarily, SLHF has been processed from mass equations that utilization ship-or ground-based estimations. Be that as it may, because of the low transient and spatial goals of this point-type information, the accessibility and exactness of station-inferred motions are moderately constrained (Singh *et al.*, 2001). By acclimatizing land surface, deliver, raw in sunder, air ship, remote detecting information and other accessible information, the NCEP/NCAR (National Centers for Environmental Prediction/National Center for (Atmospheric Research) Reanalysis System gives worldwide coordinated reanalysis information arrangement at a precision of 10– 30 W m−2, reasonable for long haul studies (1979 and fresher information – the third period of the development of the worldwide watching framework, for example the "cutting edge satellite period"). The information utilized in this paper was downloaded from the FTP Server ftp://ftp.cdc.noaa.gov. Every day SLHF data are shown by a Gaussian matrix of 94 lines from 88.542° S to 88.542° N, with ordinary 1.875° longitudinal dispersing and anticipated onto a rectangular framework (Kalnay *et al.*, 1996; Kistler *et al.*, 2001). Relating NCEP lattice esteems can be determined from the longitude and scope of individual earth-shudder epicenters (allude the last segment of Table 1).

Method

Classification of Parameters

To assess the connection between's seismic action and SLHF oddities measurably, we expected their practices' to be two free occasions and grouped their connection ships into four classifications: 00, 01, 10 and 11. To our worries, just inconsistencies that happened inside a predetermined time window before a given seismic movement were considered. Figure 2 demonstrates the four sorts of association in the territory of the Tohoku seismic action over a time of in excess of 20 yr. Speck means "day of all out years", which ranges from 1 January 1991 (DOT = 1) to 1 January 2012 (DOT = 4383). Dull triangles mark esteems that outperform the inconsistency edge, which could be translated as irregular signs. The bolts demonstrate explicit seismic movement amid the investigation time frame. As the "00" class shows a time of no seismicity or inconsistencies, just classifications "01", "10" and "11" are talked about in the accompanying segments

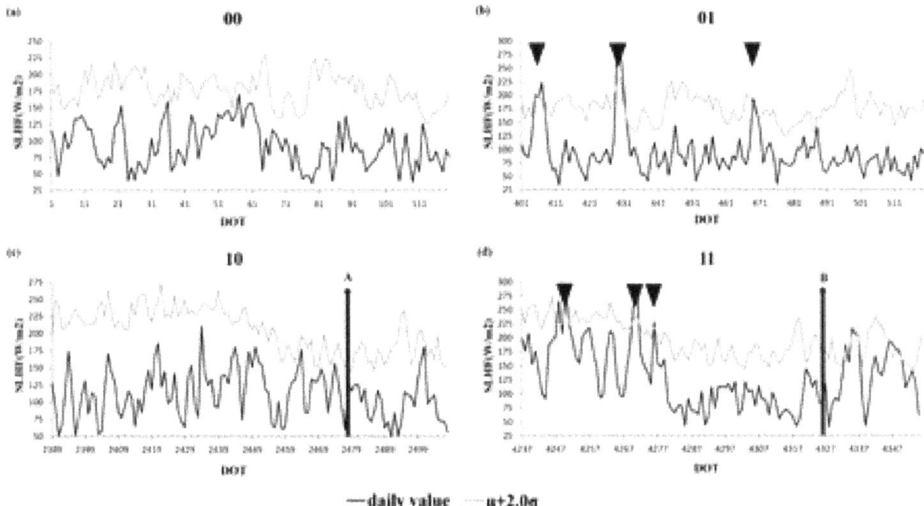

Fig 2: A shows seismic action A (15 October 1990, Mw = 6.5, 92.249° E, 2.211° S), B demonstrates seismic movement 394 B (8 November 1995, Mw = 6.8, 95.050° E, 1.833° N).

Establishment of Parameters

To characterize the warm inconsistency exactly, we right off the bat chosen four customizable parameters before the formal assessing method: (1) M -a seismic movement with a size M (Mw) or bigger is incorporated into the seismic action list and is considered for relationship examination; (2) abnormality limit – values past this edge are considered as peculiarities; (3) time window – the length of days between the start of an oddity and a seismic action; and (4) E – the degree/abundance of a bizarre esteem. For SLHF information, the unit of E is W m−2. Besides, for these seismic action, the estimations of previous two parameters were for starters fixed by past inquires about. A far reaching survey of the writing on the distinguishing proof of warm irregularities, combined with information of seismology and measurements, proposes that: (1) the parameter M can be set at a greatness of 5.0, which is a decently estimated seismic action; and (2) the peculiarity edge can be characterized as the mean estimation of SLHF information more than several years, including the investigation time frame, in addition to 2.0 occasions the standard deviation (for example $\mu + 2.0\sigma$). Thirdly, considering the different geographical and climatic foundations of these six seismic movements considered here, the estimations of time window, ΔDOT and E were built up dependent on the present moment SLHF varieties relating to each seismic action.

The variety in SLHF for 90 days preceding and 30 days following every principle stun is shown in Fig. 3. The upper dim line demonstrates the reference greatest qualities (for example irregularity edges). The lower dark line speaks to the day by day estimations of NCEP-SLHF lattice focuses enveloping the epicenter of each seismic action.

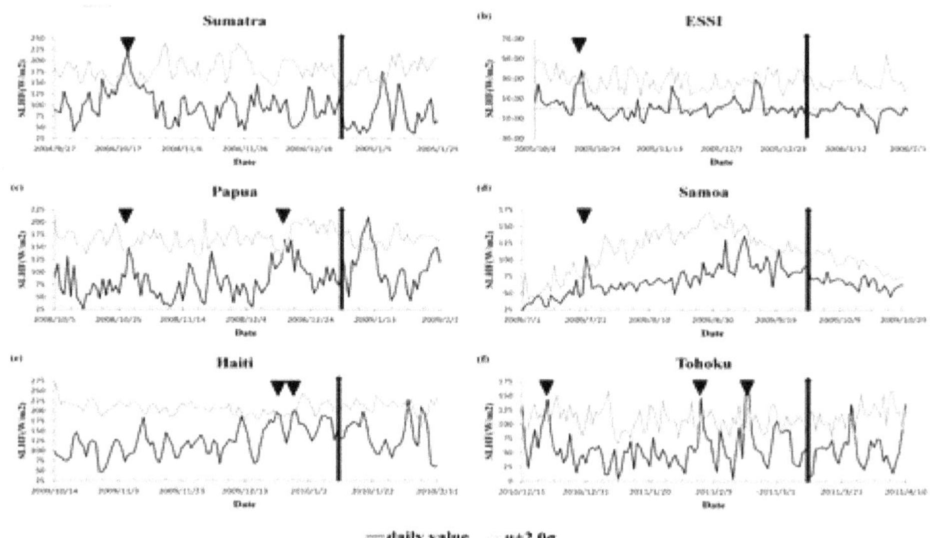

Fig 3: SHLF variation for six seismic events

The strong dark bolt shows the date of each seismic action and the triangle features SLHF irregularities. For the Sumatra seismic action, there was just a single inconsistency 69 days before the primary stun. This irregularity went on for 6 days and has a normal estimation of 22.79 W m−2. Contrasted with the oddity before the Sumatra seismic action, the abnormality related with the ESSI earth-tremor was less critical; it kept going just 2 days and had a mean estimation of 7.77 W m−2.However, given the abundance of the SLHF varieties in the ESSI region, this oddity is as yet striking. The two oddities before the Papua seismic action are hard to distinguish, and both have low ΔDOT and strange extents. Strangely, an abnormality happened 7 days after the principle stun, which was close to the pinnacle an incentive for the three months adjusting the fundamental stun. In any case, we just spotlight on preliminary SLHF abnormalities and don't examine this inconsistency further. Seventy days before the Samoa seismic action, there was one clear oddity that proceeded into the following day and found the middle value of 18.04 W m−2, which is generally huge. Two pinnacles happened before the Haiti seismic movement, however they are both little. Three pinnacles surpass the foundation level before the Tohoku seismic action. The mean estimations of these abnormalities are bigger than 30 W m−2, surpassing its $\mu + 2.0\sigma$ limit by almost 200 %. For every principle stun, the estimations of time window and ΔDOT are the greatest, while E is the normal of irregularity esteems.

Identification and Long Haul Assessing

In view of the parameters built up before in this paper, the long haul examination for related SLHF varieties and seismicity was done in two phases of correlation: "01" versus "11" and "10" versus "11". In the primary stage, we figured the probabilities of "01" and "11" happening, for example we determined the occasions that preliminary changes in SLHF fulfilled the models of being an oddity and the likelihood of seismic movement that happened inside the given time window. The varieties in SLHF inside one NCEP framework cell may be influenced by a few components, including regular changes, rainstorm, and seismic movement. To evaluate the effect of seismic action close to the epicentral NCEP framework region, all seismic action bigger than a given size (M) and inside a zone of roughly 1 million km2 around the epicenter of every one of the six seismic action (generally 10◦ longitude by 10◦ scope; the individual zone changes with the scope of every epicenter) were thought about. The domino impact of this examination is given in Table 2. To expel the foreshock-primary stun consequential convulsion impact and its effect on later changes in SLHF, we likewise joined seismic action inside 30 days of one another (alluded to as solo seismic movement).

Table 2: Gives the probabilities of "01" and "11" situations of associations between SLHF peculiarities and seismic action.

Name	Study period	Study area	No of AN	No of EQ	"01" %	"11" %
Sumatra	1 Jan 1984 – 31 Dec 2003	2 - 8◦ N, 90– 100◦ E	81	251	22.2	77.8
ESSI	1 Jan 1985– 31 Dec 2004	56 - 66◦ S, 17– 27◦ W	100	375	12.0	88.0
Papua	1 Jan 1984– 31 Dec 2003	4 - 5◦ N, 127– 137◦ E	77	61	56.0	44.0
Samoa	1 Jan 1989– 31 Dec 2008	9 -20◦ S,167 -177◦ W	86	866	9.3	90.7
Haiti	1 Jan 1989– 31 Dec 2008	13–23◦ N, 67– 77◦ W	42	31	92.9	7.1
Tohoku	1 Jan 1990– 31 Dec 2009	33– 43◦N,137–147◦ E	149	998	2.7	97.3

There are numerous occurrences in which the SLHF esteem outperformed the inconsistency limit. Haiti had the least peculiarities. All things considered, it had 42 strange varieties in the course of the last 20 yr. Before the expulsion of the seismic movement bunching impact, The quantities of seismic movement bigger than M for every one of the six cases were amazing extensive. Aside from Haiti, the rates of "11" situations were huge, demonstrating that numerous seismic movement happened after SLHF inconsistencies. After the de-bunching process, both the quantity of seismic action and the level of "11" situations diminished altogether, and the connection is factually immaterial (see Table 3).

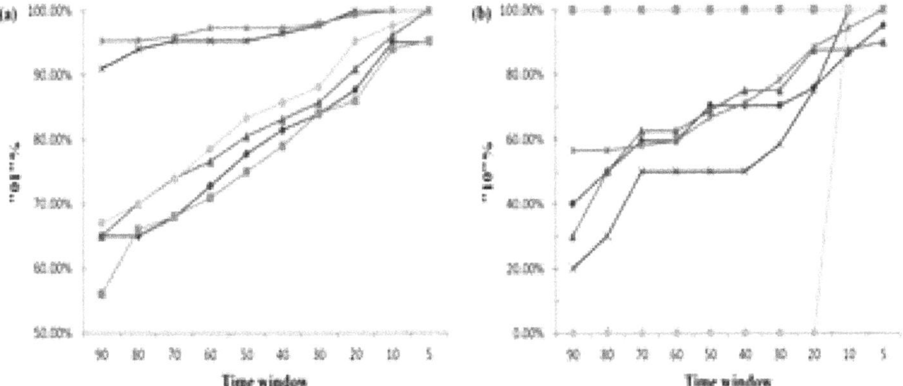

Fig 4: The association between time window and level of "01"/"10" % situations

Look at the normal estimations of SLHF. Which were no identified with the peculiarities before these seismic movement (for example "01"), it demonstrates that the unique pinnacles past to the ESSI, Samoa and Haiti seismic movement are numerically unessential. The estimations of E for ESSI, Samoa and Haiti in present moment were progressively 7.77, 18.04 and 11.48, while in long haul were 9.57, 26.17 and 17.04. As it were, these SLHF vacillations at such degrees might be typical for these regions.

Table 3: Probabilities of "01" and "11" after de - bunching.

	Sumatra	ESSI	Papua	Samoa	Haiti	Tohoku
No. of solo EQ	37	31	28	3	22	4
"01"%	67.9%	66.1%	74.1%	95.2%	95.3%	95.4%
"11"%	32.1%	34.2%	26.1%	4.71%	4.81%	4.69%
Average value (W m−2)	19.39	9.57	20.21	26.17	17.04	23.75

Discussion

Data Relevance

Despite the fact that the utilization of a homogeneous dataset (for example NCEP-SLHF) would have lightened the mistake because of various SLHF perceptions, the NCEP dataset contains assimilative information whose precision depends on a few elements. The exactness of a solitary variable at various periods changes relying upon the first information gathering strategy. Despite the fact that the NCEP reanalysis information osmosis framework is steady, the watching framework has developed generously after some time. The advancement of the worldwide watching framework is separated into three noteworthy stages: the "early" period from the 1940s through the International Geophysical Year in 1957, when the principal upper-air perceptions were made; the "cutting edge raw in sunder arrange" from 1958 to 1978; and the "cutting edge satellite time" from 1979 to the present (Kalnay *et al.*, 1996). Along these lines, the precision of reanalyzed surface inert warmth transitions is normally time-subordinate. Given the development of information exactness, the SLHF peculiarities going before the ESSI, Papua and Haiti seismic action were estimated utilizing less precise NCEP-SLHF information Therefore, these varieties may not be genuine oddities Since the historical backdrop of NCEP information is exceptionally short contrasted and the seismic action inventory, the date of a given seismic action ought to be considered before utilizing the NCEP/NCAR information in the investigation of SLHF varieties preceding seismic movement. The yield factors in NCEP/NCAR information are characterized into four classes, contingent upon the degree to which they are impacted by the observational information and additionally the digestion demonstrate. Lamentably, surface transitions are among the "C" factors, which implies that they depend vigorously on the model amid information digestion (issue to the as recreation of different perceptions) and ought to be utilized with alert (Kistler *et al.*, 2001). On the off chance that the model and its physical parameterizations are practical, the SLHF information can give air conditioning clergyman gauges, even on a day by day time scale. Notwithstanding, it will be provincially one-sided if the model is one-sided. Consequently, the model attainability ought to be checked before utilizing SLHF information from NCEP/NCAR to ponder any SLHF varieties in a particular territory.

Summary and Conclusion

In light of these assessment results got from this examination, a few ends can be drawn: (1) albeit some SLHF varieties may outperform the foundation shifting dimension, despite everything they can't be perceived as warm abnormalities as indicated by their small outperforming amplitudes and SLHF information precision; (2) the grouping impact of seismic movement succession ought to be given enough consideration amid the assessment of association between SLHF varieties and seismic action; (3) the relationship of SLHF inconsistency and seismic action is moderately low (because of shot) and to a great extent relies upon a few elements including information and parameter. We unequivocally prescribe that standard SLHF inconsistency recognizing criteria ought to be built up. While a few acclimations to parameters at the learning stage are acknowledge capable, one must guarantee that the comparing criteria have been obviously set and carefully utilized before any marvel is formally characterized as an antecedent. Regardless of whether the geo-physical hypothesis isn't seen completely, foreordained distinguishing and breaking down methods still should be considered and tended to In view of the above discoveries; a lot further work can be successfully completed. We will perform more assessments on a few other related warm parameters which are inferred by remote detecting or absorption innovation. Other related elements incorporating the regular varieties in wind and sea ebb and flow, local saltiness focus and relative moistness will be considered. In addition, keeping the benefit of remote detecting information in spatial goals as a main priority, further long haul spatial examination for the referenced seismic movement will be done. Like one single NCEP framework examination, parameters, for example, time window and oddity limit will be chosen to contemplate the spatial and fleeting association between seismic action and warm varieties. More information mining innovations will likewise add to the accompanying work.

Reference

Bourras, D.: Comparison of five satellite-inferred inactive warmth transition items to moored float information, *J. Atmosphere,* 19, 6291– 6313, doi:10.1175/JCLI3977.1, 2006.

Cervone, G., Kafatos, M., Napoletani, D., and Singh, R. P.: Wavelet maxima bends of SLHF related with two late Greek seismic action, Nat. Risks *Earth Syst. Sci.*, 4, 359– 374, doi:10.5194/nhess-4-359-2004, 2004.

Cervone, G., Singh, R. P., Kafatos, M., and Yu, C.: Wavelet maxima bends of surface dormant warmth motion oddities related with Indian seismic action, Nat. Dangers Earth Syst. Sci., 5,87– 99, doi:10.5194/nhess-5-87-2005, 2005.

Chen, M., Deng, Z., Yang, Z., and Ma, X.: SLHF irregularities before the Indonesia Mw 9.0 seismic movement of 2004, Chinese Sci. Bull., 51, 1010– 1013, doi: 10.1007/s11434-006-1010-y, 2006.

Choudhury, S., Dasgupta, S., Saraf, A. K., and Panda, S.: Remote detecting perceptions of pre-seismic action warm abnormalities in Iran, *Int. J. Remote Sens.*, 27, 4381– 4396, doi: 10.1080/01431160600851827, 2006.

Freund, F. T., Takeuchi, A., Lau, B. W. S., Al-Manaseer, A., Fu, C. C., Bryant, N. An., and Ouzounov, D.: Stimulated infrared discharge from rocks: surveying a pressure pointer, eEarth,2, 7– 16, doi:10.5194/ee-2-7-2007, 2007.

Innovations in Biochemical Techniques (2020) : Page no. 81-103
ASTRAL INTERNATIONAL (P) LTD., New Delhi - 110002

Chapter 7

Production, Optimization and Partial Purification of Detergent Compatible and Thermostable Alkaline Protease by *Bacillus clausii* PHBS 12A

Jayarathne J.A.J.C., Dahal K., Mukherjee M. and Prakash P

The Oxford College of Science, No.32, 17th B Main, Sector IV, HSR Layout, Bengaluru 560102, Karnataka, India E-mail: pathangep@gmail.com

Abstract

Microbial proteases are hydrolytic enzymes widely used in many industrial processes and management of wastes. This study was conducted with the aim of screening for efficient protease-producing bacteria from soils and agro-industrial wastes, determining optimal production conditions and partially characterizing the stability and activity of the protease with regards to some physicochemical parameters. The bacterium used in this study was the strain of PHBS isolated and identified earlier as *Bacillus clausii*. The optimum protease production time was found to be 48 h corresponding to a protease activity of 30 U/ml. The optimum temperature of protease production was 37°C, corresponding to 32.2 U/ml. Among the various carbon sources tested, sucrose gave the maximum activity (30.4 U/ml) and regarding nitrogen sources, casein gave maximum activity (36.1 U/ml). Furthermore, 0.6 M NaCl concentrations were found to give better protease production than the media containing no NaCl. Studies on the effect of pH on the activity and stability of protease enzymes revealed that the crude enzyme had a maximum activity and stability at pH 11. These results generally indicate that the proteases obtained in this study belong to the class of alkaline protease. Furthermore, the evaluation of some agro-industrial wastes as potential substrates for protease production indicated that corn husk and chicken feathers were better.

Keywords: *Bacillus sp., casein hydrolysis, enzyme activity, protease, soil, agro-industrial wastes.*

Introduction

Enzymes are highly efficient and environmentally friendly protein catalysts synthesized by living systems. They are characterized by specificity, high catalytic activity, and ability to work at moderate as well as extreme temperatures. Enzymes are well-known biocatalysts that perform a multitude of chemical reactions and are commercially exploited in the detergent, food, pharmaceutical, diagnostics, and fine chemical industries.

Proteases are a large group of proteolytic enzymes that are ubiquitous in nature. They are involved in the regulation of metabolism and gene expression, enzyme modification, pathogenicity, and the hydrolysis of large proteins to smaller molecules for transport and metabolism (Rao *et al.*, 1998).

The extracellular proteases are of commercial value and find multiple applications in various industrial sectors. Proteases are obtained from plant, animal and microbial sources (Gupta *et al.*, 2002).

In the last 30 years, different classes of proteases of commercial importance have been produced from microbial, animal and plant sources and implemented for enormous applications in a range of processes that take advantage of the unique physical and catalytic properties of individual proteolytic enzyme types. Proteases from microbial sources possess almost all the characteristics desired for their biotechnological applications (Rao *et al.*, 1998).

With increasing industrial demands for biocatalysts that can cope with the industrial processes at harsh conditions, the isolation and characterization of new promising strains are possible ways to increase the diversity and yield of such enzymes (Gupta *et al.*, 2002).

The proteases available today in the market are derived from microbial sources. Most of the commercially important alkaline proteases are produced by Bacillus spp. The alkaline proteases derived pH and temperature ranges, broad substrate-specific, and can be easily purified with low cost (Haddar *et al.*, 2009). This is due to their high productivity, limited cultivation space requirement, easy genetic manipulation, broad biochemical diversity and desirable characteristics that make them suitable for biotechnological applications (Genckal, 2004; Singhal *et al.*, 2012). Proteases are ubiquitous and found in several microorganisms such as protozoa, bacteria, yeast and fungi.

As acknowledged the Bacillus sp. are well known for the production of extracellular protease. Most bacteria from the Bacillus species can be obtained from soil and are preferred to be used in the production of extracellular enzymes. As the title of the research implies, the aim is to produce extracellular protease, therefore, any mesophilic bacterium in the genus Bacillus is favorable in terms of extracellular proteases (Abdullah, 2006). The detergent industry requires efficient, environmentally friendly and economical strategies for unwanted protein degradation. Alkaline proteases in detergent formulations can act against proteinaceous stains like blood, food and grass stains (Hameed *et al.*, 1996; Smulders *et al.*, 2002; Huang *et al.*, 2003; Wang *et al.*, 2007; Devi *et al.*, 2008).

Proteases find huge potential in various food and feed industrial applications such as in dairy industry (milk protein; casein and whey protein hydrolysis for use in cheese flavor development), baking industry (treatment of flour in the manufacture of baked goods and improvement of dough texture, flavour, and colour in cookies, *etc.*), brewing industry, soy protein hydrolysis, soy sauce production, gelatin hydrolysis, meat protein recovery, fish protein hydrolysis and meat tenderization and improves digestibility of animal feeds (Gupta *et al.*,2002; Sumantha *et al.*, 2006; Ikram, 2008; Nadeem, 2009).

The conventional methods in leather processing involve the use of hydrogen sulfide and other chemicals, creating environmental pollution and safety hazards. Thus, for environmental reasons, the biotreatment of leather using an enzymatic approach is preferable as it offers several advantages, *e.g.* easy control, speed and waste reduction, thus being eco-friendly. Proteases find their use in the soaking, dehairing and bating stages of preparing skins and hides. Alkaline protease with elastolytic and keratinolytic activity has been used in leather-processing industries.

Alkaline proteases speed up the process of dehairing, because the alkaline conditions enable the swelling of hair roots; and the subsequent attack of protease on the hair follicle protein allows easy removal of the hair (Gupta, *et al*; 2002a; Genckal, 2004; Ikram, 2008; Nadeem, 2009; Ray, 2012).

Alkaline proteases play a crucial role in the bioprocessing of used X-ray or photographic films for silver recovery. Conventionally, this silver is recovered by burning the films, which causes undesirable environmental pollution. Furthermore, the base film made of polyester cannot be recovered using this method. Since the silver is bound to gelatin, it is possible to extract silver from the protein layer by proteolytic treatments. Proteolytic hydrolysis of gelatin not only helps in extracting silver but also the polyester film base can be recycled (Gupta *et al*; 2002a; Genckal, 2004; Nadeem, 2009; Ray, 2012).

The global environment is gradually deteriorating because of the socio-economic activities of humankind such as processing industries. Many industrial processes cause adverse changes in the immediate environmental change and therefore being challenged by society. Of these, leather industries and the increased amount of feathers generated by commercial poultry processing may represent a pollution problem and needs adequate management. In this regard, the use of alkaline protease in the management of wastes from various industries and household activities opened up a new era in the use of proteases in waste management. Proteases solubilize proteinaceous waste and thus help lower the biological oxygen demand of aquatic systems. Alkaline protease from B. subtilis was used for the management of waste feathers from poultry slaughterhouses (Gupta, *et al*; 2002a; Genckal, 2004; Ikram, 2008; Nadeem, 2009; Ray, 2012). Although industrially applicable protease enzymes have been identified from different sources, most of them could not resist drastic environmental changes and most of the sources are incapable to produce required quantities to fulfill industrial demands. So, new bacterial strains that can withstand harsh environmental conditions should be isolated for the enhanced production of such enzymes. The present study is aimed at the isolation of a proteolytic strain from soil biome and optimization of its cultural conditions for the enhanced enzyme production.

Materials and Methods

Screening of the Organism

Casein Hydrolysis Test

Those colonies that were able to hydrolyze gelatin were further inoculated on nutrient agar containing 1% casein (w/v) and incubated at 37°C for 24 hours. Casein hydrolysis was visualized by the application of 30% trichloroacetic acid on the agar surface. A transparent halo around the bacterial growth was considered as being a positive reaction.

Assay of Protease

The bacteria was inoculated into medium consisting of 1% glucose, 0.5% peptone, 0.2% yeast extract, 0.1%K2HPO4 and 0.02% MgSO4 and incubated at 37°C. The culture broth was centrifuged at 10000 rpm for 15 min at 4°C and used as the enzyme source for quantitative studies.

Protease activity was determined using casein as a substrate.The reaction mixture contained a total volume of 2 ml which in turn was composed of 1 ml of 1% casein in 50 mM sodium phosphate buffer (pH 7) and 1 ml enzyme solution. After 20 min of incubation at 37°C, the reaction was terminated by adding 2 ml of 10% trichloroacetic acid (TCA) and again incubated at 37°C for 20 min. After separation of the un-reacted casein precipitated by centrifugation at 10000 rpm for 15 min, 0.5 ml of clear supernatant was mixed with 2.5 ml of 0.5M Na_2CO_3 and 0.5 ml of 1N Folin-Ciocalteau's phenol reagent. After incubation for 20 min at 37°C, absorbance was measured at 660 nm against a reagent blank. One unit of protease activity was defined as the amount of enzyme that releases 1 μg amino acid equivalent to tyrosine per min under the standard assay conditions (Hema and Shiny, 2012; Sevinc and Demirkan, 2011).

Production of Protease

For enzyme production, bacterial cells from a 24 h aged culture were inoculated into 100 ml Erlenmeyer flasks containing 50 ml of sterile inoculation medium containing 1% glucose, 0.5% peptone, 0.2% yeast extract, 0.1% K_2HPO_4 and 0.02% MgSO4 was inoculated with 1ml of pure culture and incubated at different temperatures, pH conditions, NaCl concentrations.

Optimization of the Growth Conditions for Production of Protease

Effect of Time on the Production of Protease

To determine the time for maximum production of protease, the 24 h growth isolate was inoculated into the medium as before and incubate at 37°C for 24-60. Two ml of the sample from the medium was collected every 12 h to determine protease activity.

Effect of Temperature on the Production of Protease

The optimum temperature for protease production was determined by incubating the culture at different temperatures (i.e. 30, 37, 40, 45 and 50°C), at pH 7 for 36 h. At the end of the incubation period, the cell-free culture filtrate was tested for protease activity using the method described above.

Effect of pH on the Production of Protease

The effect of pH on the production of protease was investigated by adjusting the pH of the growth medium to pH 5.0, 6.0, 7.0, 8.0, and 9.0 and incubating at 37°C for 36 h. The adjustment of pH was done using 1N NaOH and 0.1N HCl solutions. At the end of the incubation period, the protease activity was determined as mentioned before.

Effect of Carbon Source on the Production of Protease

Various carbon sources such as glucose, lactose, sucrose, CMC and maltose were used while keeping all other conditions the same. At the end of the incubation period, the protease activity was determined.

Effect of Nitrogen Source on the Production of Protease

Different sources of nitrogen were tested for their potentials to enhance protease production. The production medium was initially supplemented with different organic nitrogen sources such as yeast extract, peptone, and casein, each at 1% (w/v). The effect was studied by determining the protease activity.

Effect of NaCl Concentration on the Production of Protease

NaCl was added at various concentrations, i.e. 0.0, 0.2, 0.4, 0.6 and 0.8M, into the protease production medium and assay for crude enzyme (protease) activity was carried out incubating the culture for 48 h. The effect of the concentration of NaCl was studied by considering results of the protease activity, higher activity of protease was due to higher production of protease.

Use of Agro-industrial Wastes as Substrates for Protease Production

To find out the suitability of agro-industrial-based waste as a substrate for protease production, different substrates viz. corn husk, chicken feathers were tested by replacing carbon and nitrogen sources for isolates in the growth media under SMF (Submerged Fermentation). The enzyme activity was measured after 48-hour growth for the determination of protease production.

Partial Purification

Cell-free supernatant was precipitated by adding ammonium sulfate at 60% saturation level After each addition, the enzyme solution was stirred for 1 h at 4°C The protein precipitated was collected by centrifugation at 12,000 rpm for 20 min at 4C pellet was then resuspended in minimum volume of 0.05M glycine NaOH buffer pH 11Enzyme suspension was dialyzed against the same buffer with 4-6 changes.

Characterization of Protease

Effect of pH on the Activity and Stability of Protease

The dialyzed protease was incubated at different pH values such as 5, 6, 7, 8, 9, and 10 with phosphate buffer (pH 7.0). The effect on the activity was studied by incubating for 20 min and determining the remaining activity following the standard protease assay procedures described above. The effect on the stability was studied by pre-incubating for 12 hours and determining the remaining activity following the standard protease assay procedures.

Effect of Temperature on the Activity and Stability of Protease

This experiment was performed by incubating dialyzed protease at different temperatures viz.: 30, 40, and 50 60, 65, 70, 75 and 80°C. The effect on the activity was studied by incubating for 20 min and determining the remaining activity following the standard protease assay procedures described above. The effect on the stability was studied by pre-incubating for 12 hours and determining theremaining activity following the standard protease assay procedures.

Effect of Divalent Ions on the Activity of Protease

The effects of Ca^{2}+, Mg^{2}+, Mn^{2}+, Fe^{2}+ and Zn^{2}+ ions on crude protease extract were investigated by adding these cations to the reaction mixture to final concentrations of 1 mm. Enzyme activities in all cases were measured under conditions of optimum pH and temperature required for activity.

Results and Discussion

Casein hydrolysis was visualized by the application of 30% trichloroacetic acid on the agar surface. A transparent halo around the bacterial growth was considered as being a positive reaction (Fig 1). On the basis of the ratio of the diameter of the zone of clearance (mm) and colony size (mm), isolate PHBS 12A displayed the highest enzyme production was selected for further screening and identification. Morphological and cultural characteristics revealed that the isolate PHBS 12 A was gram-positive, endospore-forming rods. The growth of isolate PHBS 12A on nutrient agar was as large, irregular, flat, rough, cream and opaque colonies. The isolate was further identified described as Bacillus Clausii PHBS 12A based on 16S rDNA gene sequencing and deducing phylogenic identity.

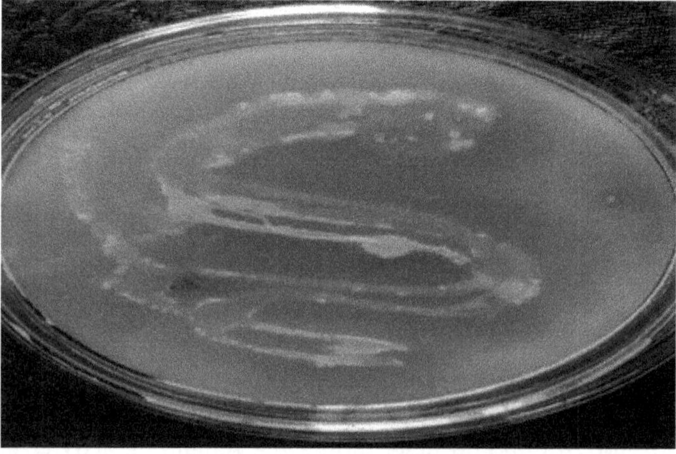

Fig 1: Casein Hydrolysis Test

Incubation Time on Protease Production

Time course of protease production by Bacillus clausii PHBS 12A was performed under the submerged condition at 1200 rpm. The bacterium depicted little growth in 6h and entered the exponential phase after 12h where the synthesis and secretion started. The stationary phase started after 24h. In the present study, the optimum protease production time was found to be 48h corresponding to protease activity of 30 U/ml (Fig 2). A gradual decrease in enzyme units was observed with an increase in the incubation period, clearly suggesting that the enzyme production is growth associated in nature. Many researchers described the production of alkaline protease by different species of Bacillus (Sharma *et al.*, 2014, Asha and Palaniswami, 2018). Multiple studies reported that maximum protease production by Bacillus sp. at 48 to 72h of the incubation period (Hoshino *et al.*, 1995; Shumi *et al.*, 2004) not only that but also several researchers reported 48h of incubation time to be the optimal time period for many Bacillus spfor the production of protease. Optimization studies of Bacillus coagulans PSB-07 by Olajuyigbe and Ehiosun, 2013, Bacillus pumilus D-6 by Bajaj and Jamwal, 2013, Bacillus firmus by Vadlamani and Parcha, 2012 and Bacillus tequilensis strain SCSGAB0139 by Aruna *et al.*, 2014 are some of the studies which reported 48 h of optimum incubation period for maximum protease production. Ward, 1995 explained that more protease production by Bacillus sp. occurred during the late exponential phase and was correlated with the high rate of protein turnover during endospores formation. Differences in the cultivation conditions and the Bacillus sp. might have an impact on the differences in the growth rate between the previous experiments and the current findings.

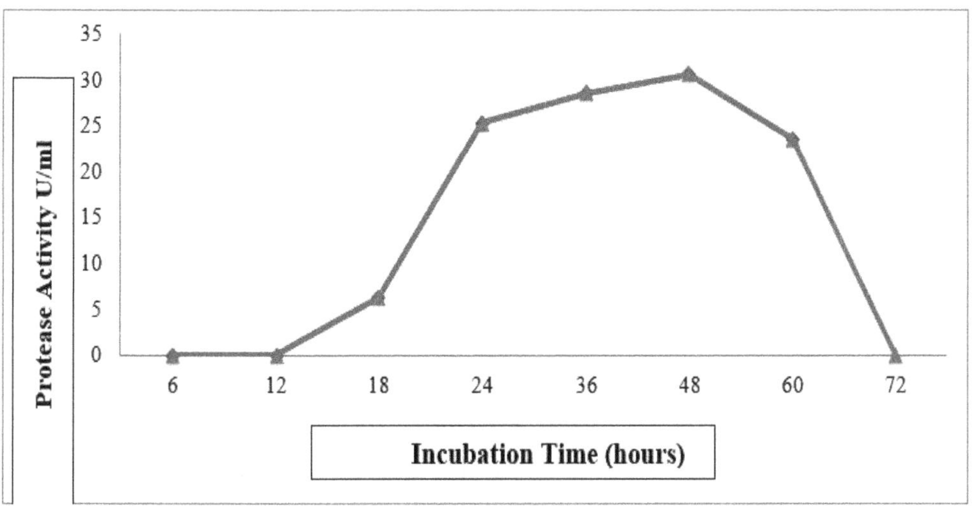

Fig 2: Effect of Incubation Time on Protease Production

Effect of Temperature on Protease Production

The optimum temperature was found to be 37°C corresponding to protease activities of 32.2 U/ml (Fig 3). Whereas, progressive decline of enzyme production was observed after their respective optimum temperatures and less enzyme production was observed up to 50°C. The above results suggested that temperature has a profound influence on the production of alkaline protease by Bacillus clausii PHBS12A. This report is very similar to the Rathod and Pathak, 2016 reported maximum alkaline protease production at 30°C by Halomonas venusta LAP515. Although the mechanism of temperature control over alkaline protease production is poorly known, it influences the synthesis and secretion of enzyme by regulating energy metabolism and oxygen uptake, by translational synthesis of protein and by altering physical properties of cell membrane of microorganisms (Frankena *et al.*, 1986, Votruba *et al.*, 1991, Rahman *et al.*, 2005). Rathod and Pathak, 2016 reported maximum alkaline protease production at 30°C by Halomonasvenusta LAP515. Although the mechanism of temperature control over alkaline protease production is poorly known maybe by altering physical properties of the cell membrane of microorganisms during the synthesis and secretion of the enzyme by regulating energy metabolism and oxygen uptake, by the translational synthesis of protein.

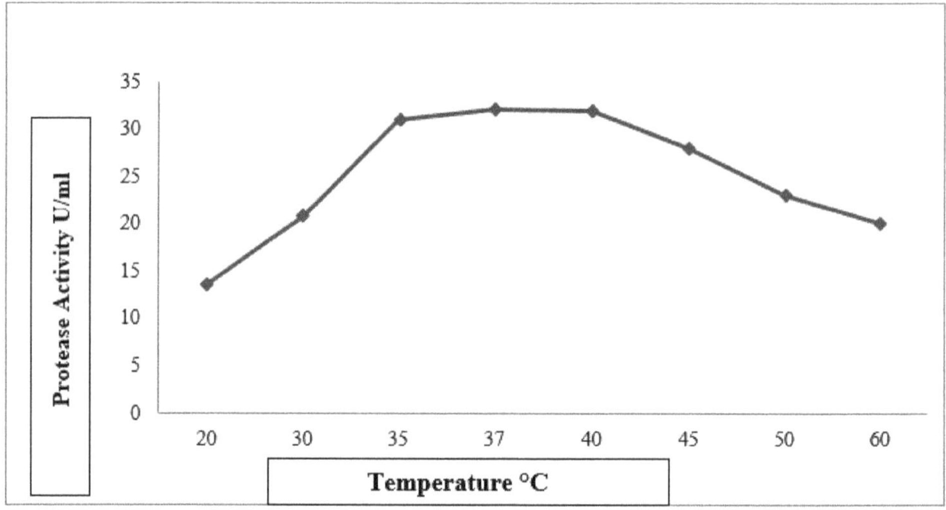

Fig 3: Effect of Temperature on Protease Production

Effect of Carbon Sources on Protease Production

Among the various carbon sources used for protease production, sucrose and lactose showed almost similar activities of 30.3 and 30.4 respectively (Fig.4). Maltose and Glucose also showed considerable activity. The enzyme production was higher compared to the commonly used carbon source glucose. Our results are in good accordance with Mabrouk *et al.*, 1999, wherein maximum enzyme production by Bacillus licheniformis ATCC 21415 was achieved in the presence of lactose or fructose. Nevertheless, Gessesse *et al.*, 2003 reported an increased level of protease production by Bacillus pseudofirmus AL-89 upon the addition of glucose, whereas the suppression of enzyme production by Nesterenkonia sp. AL-20 was obtained in the presence of glucose. According to Ibrahim *et al.*, 2015 protease production from Bacillus sp. NPST-AK15 drastically decreased in the presence of glucose and maltose. Fructose has supported maximum support. This evidence is completely deviating from our current findings. Many researchers have reported similar results like our current findings. Suganthi *et al.* 2013 reported that Bacillus licheniformis has given similar results as ours that a significant amount of protease was produced in the presence of maltose and lactose. Tambekar and Tambekar, 2013 reported a halophilic bacterium, Bacillus odysseyi, which utilized lactose as a carbon source for maximum protease production compared to fructose, maltose or starch. Other important carbon sources for protease production as reported by previous studies included glucose (Badhe *et al.*, 2016; Dorcas and Pindi, 2016) and maltose (Saraswathy *et al.*, 2013; Vanitha *et al.*, 2014).

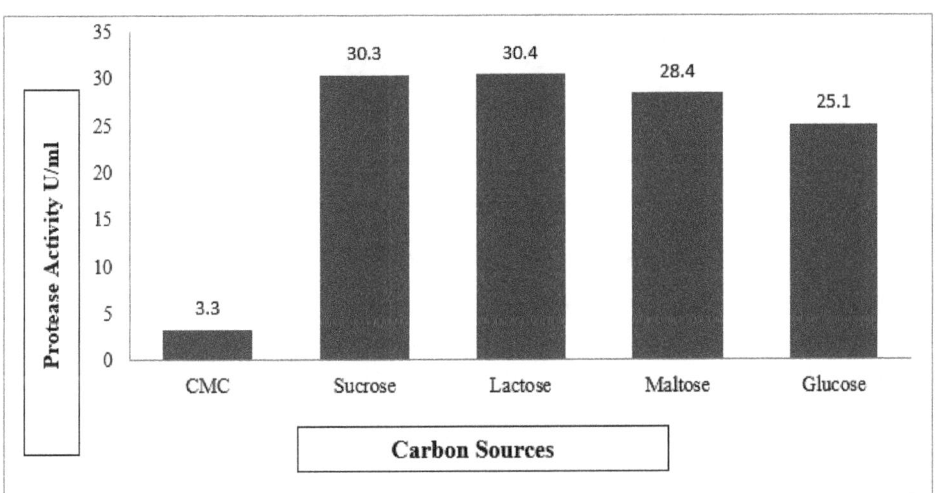

Fig 4: Effect of Carbon Sources on Protease Production

Effect of pH on Protease Production

Nutrient transport across the cell membrane and the enzymatic processes are significantly affected by the pH. The optimum pH for protease production was 11 (Fig 5). At pH 11, the protease activity was 31 U/ml. This indicates the alkaliphilic nature of the bacterial isolate. The maximum enzyme production was observed at pH 10.0(178±1.9 U ml-1) and at pH 11.0. Nevertheless, the alkaline protease production was significantly reduced at pH 5.0 and pH 12.0. Pant *et al.*, 2015 reported an optimum pH 10.0 for alkaline protease production by Bacillus subtilis. Furthermore few studies have reported similar results as our current findings. Boomindhan *et al.*, 2009 reported that Bacillus subtilis have depicted the production of protease from pH range 7 to 11 in which pH 10 was reported as the optimal pH. Sen and Sathyanarayana. 1993 reported that Bacillus licheniformis S-40 was able to grow in a pH range of 7-12 with better protease production in the alkaline range. Kumar *et al.*, 1999, Pastor *et al.*, 2001 and Khusro, 2015 demonstrated the alkaline pH optima of Bacillus sp. for protease production. However, from the survey of the literature, it can be seen that the optimum pH range for protease production is generally between pH 7 and 11 (Joo *et al.*, 2005) (Shivanand *et al.*, 2009).

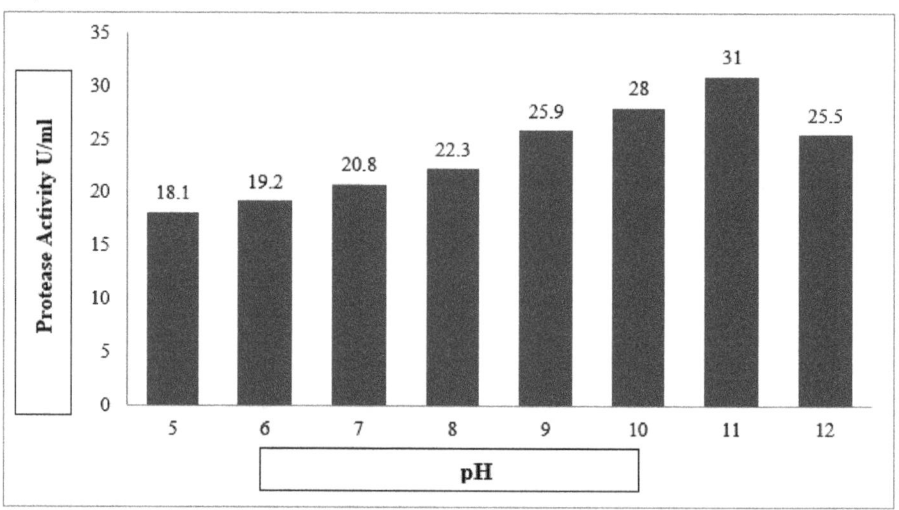

Fig 5: Effect of pH on Protease Production

Effect of Nitrogen Sources on Protease Production

Protease production is influenced by different nitrogen sources and many bacterial strains use different sources for maximum enzyme production (Gupta and Khare *et al.*, 2007). Effect of various inorganic nitrogen sources on protease production was also examined. It was observed that the growth medium containing casein yielded the highest activity of 37.2 U/ml (Fig 6). This was followed by peptone, yeast extract, potassium nitrate, ammonium sulfate and ammonium chloride. Bacillus subtilis 12A PHBS has utilized both organic and inorganic nitrogen sources and that shows the versatility of the strain to utilize numerous nitrogen sources. Pant *et al.*, 2015 reported that the utilization of casein has a significant impact on the production of protease by Bacillus subtilis sp. In addition to that many microorganismsuse casein as the major nitrogen source in maximum enzyme production. Jayasree *et al.*, (2009) reported 1% casein as the main source of nitrogen for alkaline protease production by Streptomyces pulveraceus. El Zawahry *et al.*, (2007) reported that Streptomyces halstedii Salh-12 and Streptomyces endus Salh40, two most potent proteolytic halotolerant thermophilic and mesophilic organisms respectively utilized 1% casein as a major nitrogen source in protease production medium. Different organic nitrogen sources like peptone, beef extract and yeast extract for the production of alkaline protease by Bacillus sp. have been documented by Ghafoor and Hasnain, 2009 and Marathe *et al.*, 2018.This result was in agreement with that reported for marine Bacillus sp. MIG (Sánchez *et al.*, 2003), alkaliphilic Bacillus pumilus MCAS8 (Jayakumar *et al.*, 2012), alkaliphilic Bacillus licheniformis KBDL4 (Deng *et al.*, 2010) and Bacillus cluasii (Lakshmi *et al.*, 2014) where alkaline protease production was maximal using yeast extract, and significantly reduced using inorganic nitrogen sources. In earlier reports, it was found that other organic nitrogen sources supported protease production in other microorganisms including skim milk (Faranaket *et al.*, 2008).

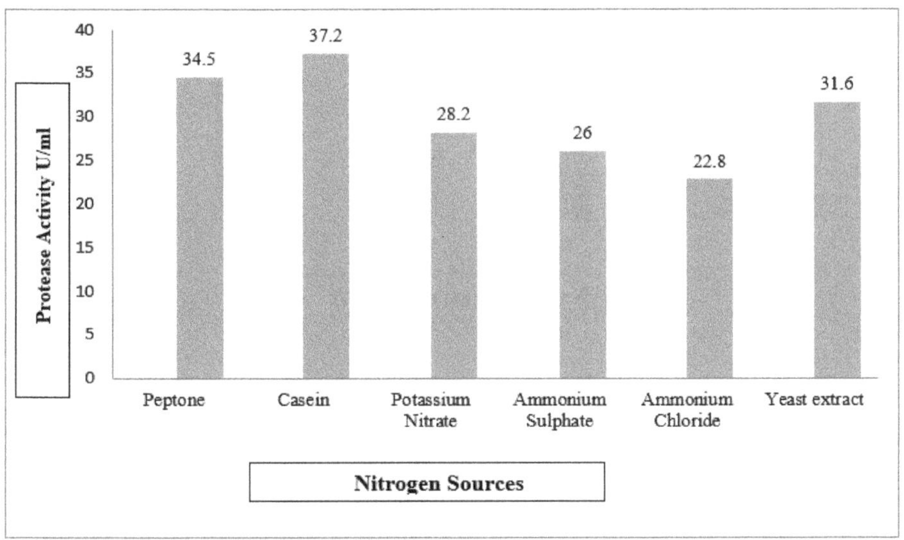

Fig 6: Effect of Nitrogen Sources on Protease Production

Effect of NaCl Concentration on the Production of Protease

Various NaCl concentrations (i.e. 0, 0.2, 0.4, 0.6, 0.8M) were used to determine optimum level required for the production of protease. It was revealed that strain Bacillus Clausii PHBS 12A can grow over a wide range of NaCl concentrations. It was observed that the growth medium containing 0.6M yielded the maximum activity of 32.5 U/ml (Fig. 7). This was followed by 0.4M of NaCl for 30.1 U/ml. It was also observed that 0.8 M NaCl concentrations resulted in the least protease production of 16.0 U/ml.However, higher NaCl concentration led to a drastic reduction in both growth and protease production. An increased concentration of salt changes the lipid composition of the cell membrane which eventually decreases the growth rate along with the enzyme production. Studies have described a reduction of enzyme production by gram-positive halophilic bacteria when the salt concentration is increased (Ventosa *et al.*, 1998). B. aquimaris by Shivanand and Jayaraman *et al.*, 2009 and B. licheniformis by Suganthi *et al.*, 2013 reported that 1M concentration of NaCl gave the maximum protease production. It clearly indicates that Bacillus Clausii PHBS 12A is halotolerant and its extracellular alkaline protease with salt tolerance signifies their potential applicability in the laundry industry in a better way than the other reported proteases from Bacillus sp.

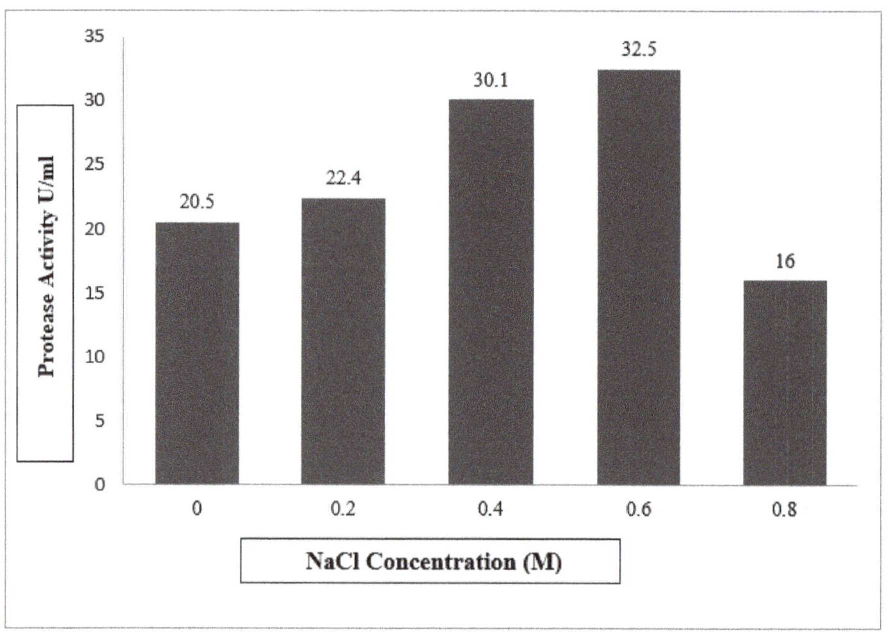

Fig 7: Effect of NaCl Concentration on the Production of Protease

Characterization of Protease

Effect of pH on the Activity of the Partially Purified Enzyme

The effect of pH on the activity of protease was studied by incubating the reaction mixture at pH values ranging from 6 to 12 and a temperature of 37°C for 20 min. The highest protease activity was shown at pH 11 (Fig. 8). These results suggest that the protease of this study belongs to the alkaline protease group. Closely similar results have been reported by Kalwasinksa *et al.*, 2018 pertaining to Bacillus luteus H11 strain.

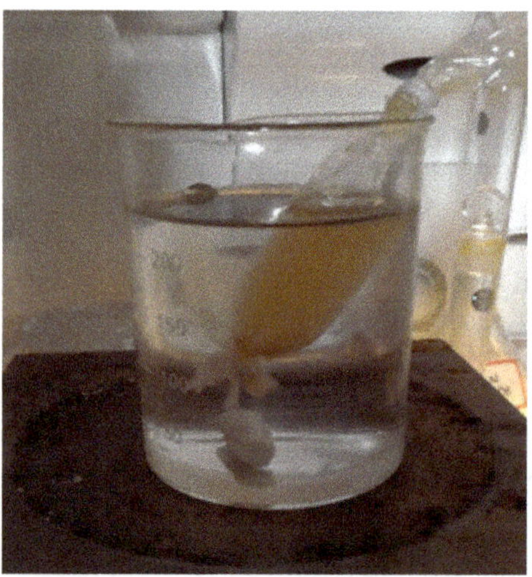

Partial Purification of Protease

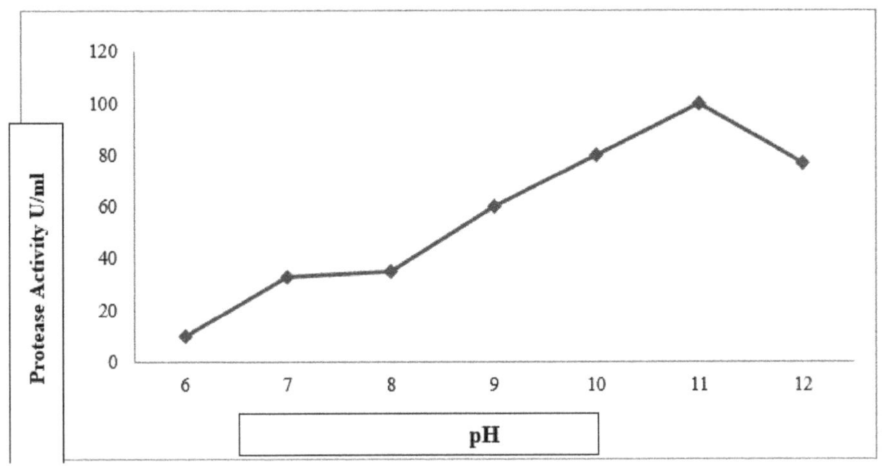

Fig 8: Effect of pH on the Activity of the Partially Purified Enzyme

Effect of pH on the Stability of Protease

The effect of pH on enzyme stability was examined by incubating the reaction mixture at pH values ranging from 6.0 to 12.0 and a temperature 37°C for 12 hours with casein in sodium phosphate buffer. The results showed that the stability of the protease was higher at pH values ranging from 8.0 to 12.0 than at lower pH values exhibiting maximum stability at pH 11(Fig. 9). These findings suggest that the proteases belonged to the alkaline protease class.

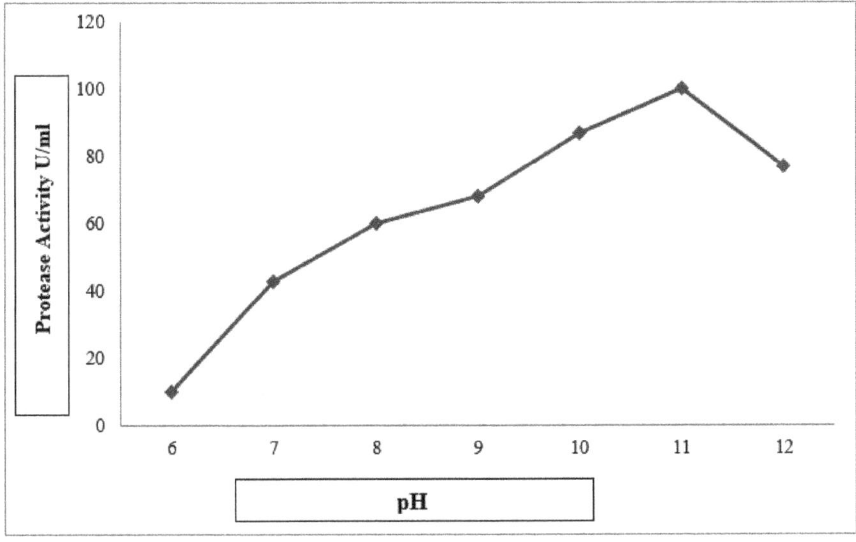

Fig 9: Effect of pH on the Stability of Protease

Effect of Incubation Temperature on the Activity of Partially Purified Protease Enzyme

The effect of temperature on the activity of protease was studied, by incubating the partially purified protease with the substrate at temperatures ranging from 20 to 80°C and at optimum pH for 20 min. The highest protease activity was for 60°C (Fig.10). The results of this study clearly indicated that the protease obtained was thermostable.

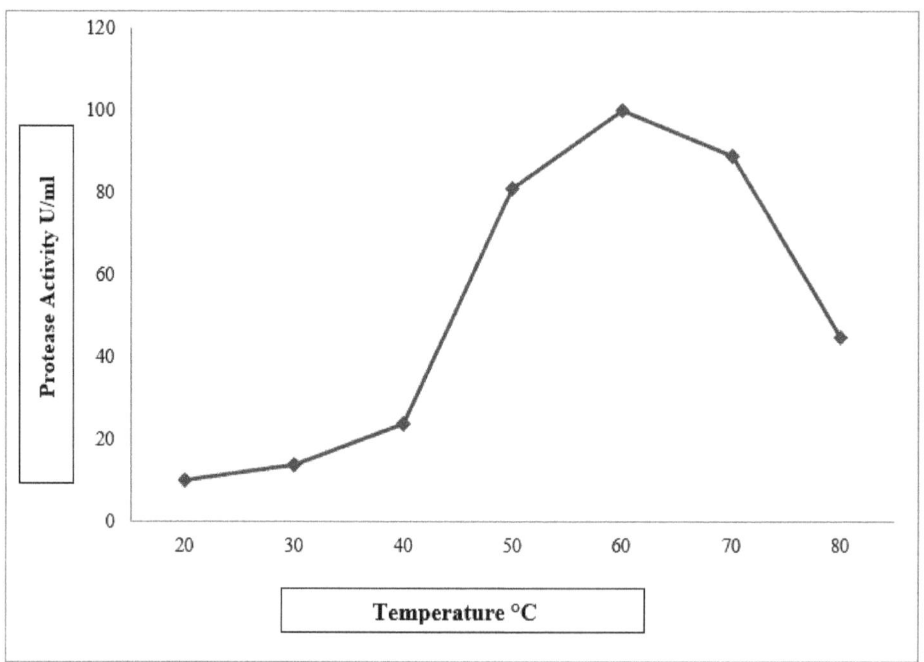

Fig 10: Effect of Incubation Temperature on the Activity of Partially Purified Protease Enzyme

Effect of Temperature on the Stability of the Partially Purified Enzyme

The effect of temperature on the stability of proteases was also measured by pre-incubating them at the optimum pH for 12h. As shown in Fig. 11, the enzyme is active after incubation at temperatures between 30 and 80°C, with the highest stability obtained when held at 60°C. The protease activity was relatively stable at temperatures ranging from 60-65°C and 85.2% of the activity was retained after incubation at 70°C. For most of the halophilic proteases, the reported stability of the temperature ranges from 37°C to 75°C (Selin *et al.*, 2014; Vidyasagar *et al.*, 2009). Our research finding showcases significant stability at a high temperature in comparison to some studies (Kalwasinksa *et al.*, 2018)

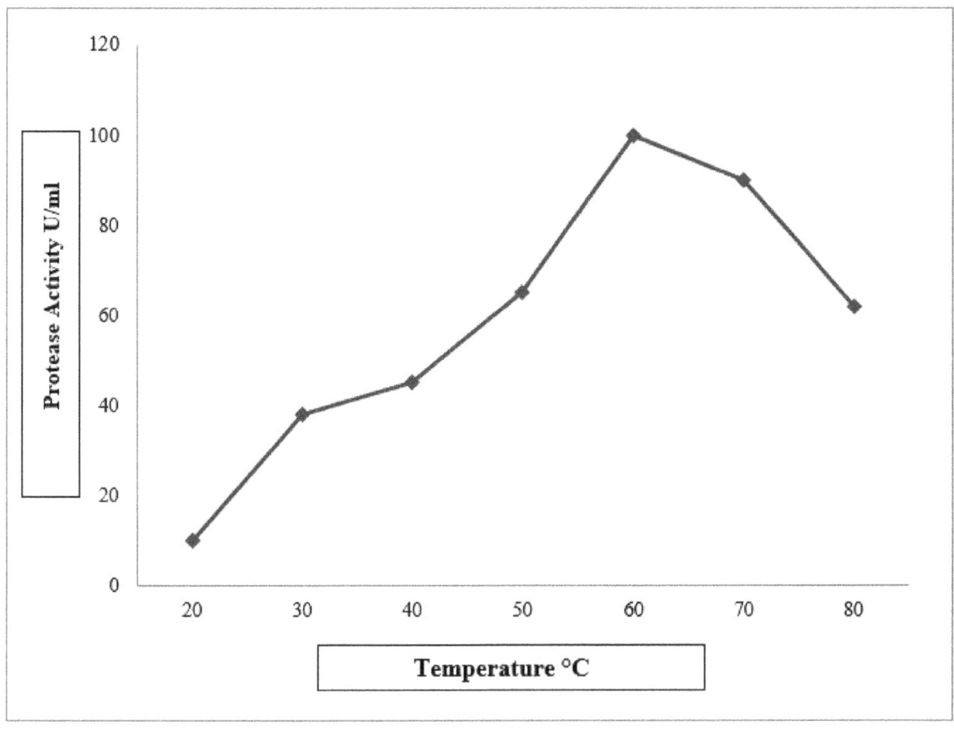

Fig 11: Effect of Temperature on the Stability of the Partially Purified Enzyme

Effect of Metallic Ions on the Activity of the Partially Purified Enzyme

The influence of metal ions on the protease activity was analyzed as shown in fig 12. The results showed that the protease was activated by Ca2+ and Mg2+ at 1mM concentration and inhibited by Zn 2+ Hg2+. Usharani and Muthuraj, 2009 described similar results pertaining to Bacillus laterosporous. It was reported that protease activity was stimulated by Ca2+ ions. This suggests that metal ions apparently protect the enzyme against thermal denaturation. Not only that but also it plays a pivotal role in maintaining the conformation of the enzyme at higher temperatures. Strong inhibitory effect by Zn 2+ and Hg2+ions are explained by Banerjee *et al.*, 1999 in Bacillus brevis. It is known that Hg2+ ions react with thiol group of protein to convert them to mercaptides (Usharani and Muthuraj, 2009) and also the action of the Hg2+ ions hydrolytically degrades the disulphide bonds (Kumar *et al.*, 1999).

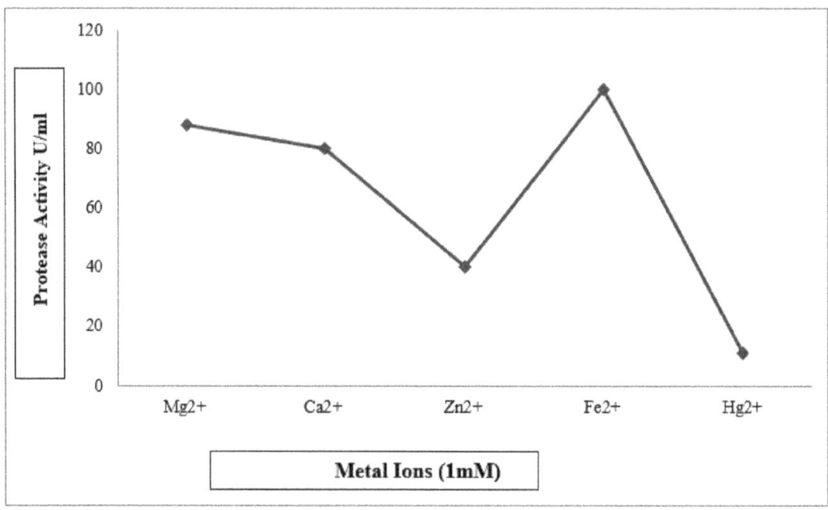

Fig 12: Effect of Metallic Ions on the Activity of the Partially Purified Enzyme

Effect of detergents (detergent compatibility)

Enzymes are used in a very small amount in detergent preparations to increase the cleaning ability of detergents. If detergent does not contain an enzyme, it may not completely remove the stains resulting in permanent residues. The performance of an enzyme in a detergent is based on the detergent composition, type of stains to be removed, water hardness, washing temperature and procedure. We used four variants of detergents available in the market and with them checked for the activity of the partially purified protease. It was found that the protease activity was not affected. Instead, it was found to be compatible with it (Fig 13). Closely similar results have been reported with respect to Bacillus sp. by Nascimento and Martinis, 2006.

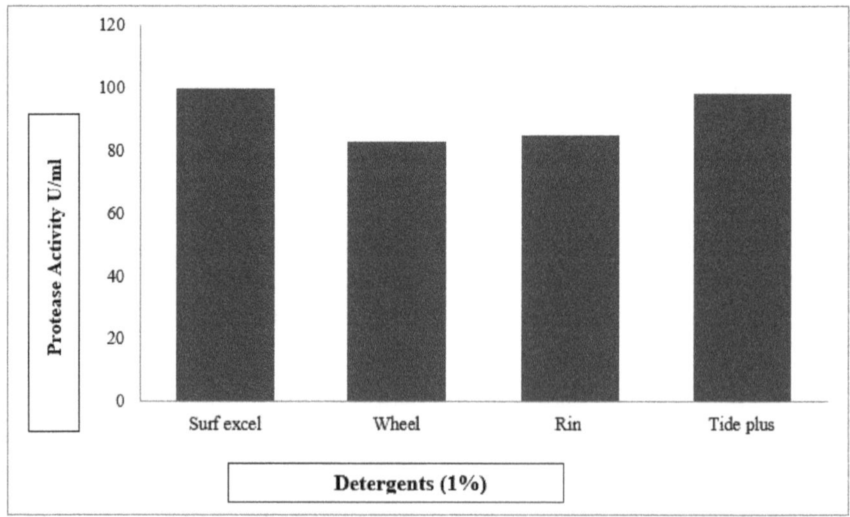

Fig 13: Effect of detergents (detergent compatibility)

Evaluation of Agro-Industrial Wastes as Sources for the Production of Protease

Evaluation of the agro-industrial wastes indicated that corn husk and chicken feathers were better for the production of protease (Fig. 14 & 15). Although microorganisms have the potential to produce enzymes, the production cost of the enzyme is the critical issue for further application at the industrial level. It is estimated that growth media accounts for 30-40% of the production cost in enzyme industries. In the present study,casein was replaced by agro wastes such as animal hairs removed from leather industries and barbershops; chicken feathers from poultry industries, corn husk, nut peel, fish scales and Sugar cane bagasse from agro-industries can serve as ideal cheap and readily available substrates. For the cost-effective commercial production of protease.

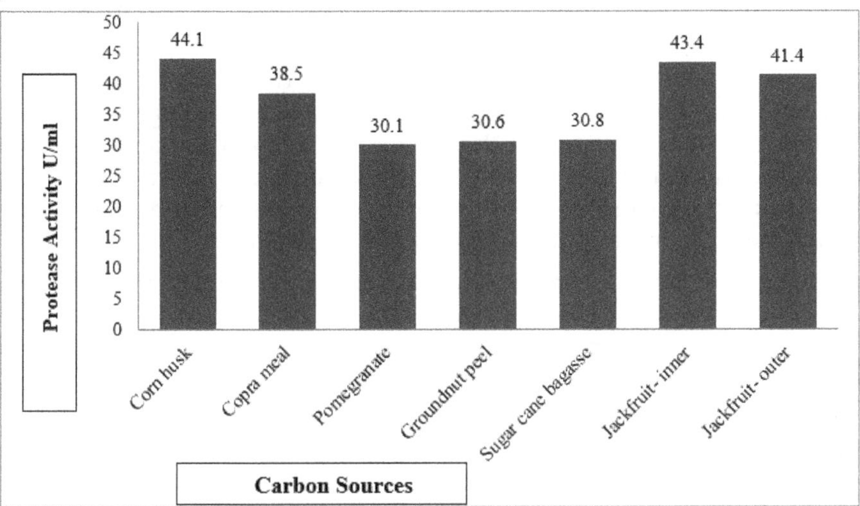

Fig 14: Different Carbon Sources on Enzyme Production

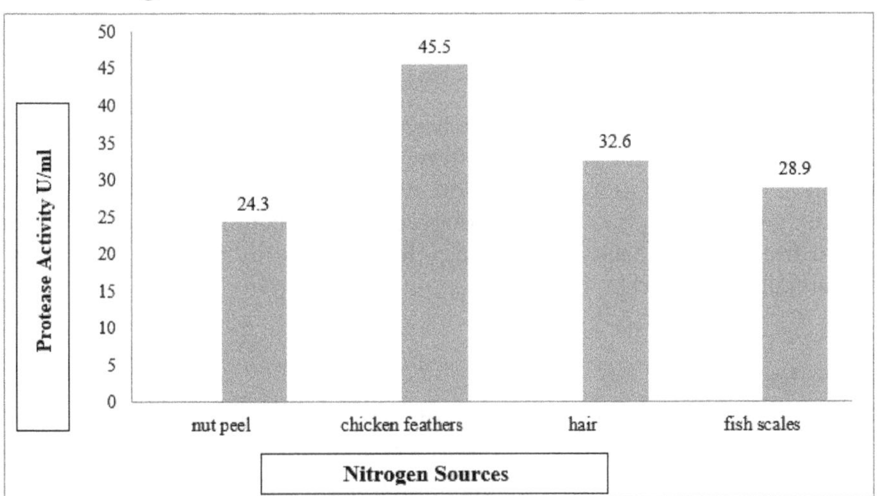

Fig 15: Different Nitrogen Sources on Enzyme Production

The results indicated that protease production varied with the type of agro-waste. Wheat bran was the best inducer for protease production with maximum protease production was observed in 1% chicken feathers after 48hours incubation, followed by hair, fish scales and nut peel.

In addition, the removal of these different Agro-industrial wastes could minimize environmental pollution.

Conclusion

Proteases are one of the most important groups of industrial enzymes with considerable application in the animal feed processing, leather industry, medical activity, beverage industry and other sectors. In this study, protease was produced by a strain of Bacillus callusi which were obtained from soil and agro-industrial wastes.

A growth media adjusted to pH 7 was used to determine the optimum time and temperature for maximum protease production. Accordingly, the optimum incubation time was found to be 48 hours at 37°C. On the other hand, the optimum temperature was found to be 37°C. Using these optimized time and temperature, the optimum pH for protease production was determined and found to be 11, although the enzyme was produced in the pH range of 6-12.

Among the various carbon sources, sucrose showed maximum enzyme production, better than glucose. Evaluation of the effect of nitrogen sources revealed that the growth medium containing casein produced maximum protease. The optimum NaCl concentration was found to be 0.6 M.

The study on the effect of pH on enzyme activity and stability showed that the protease was more active over the pH range 8.0 to 12.0, but exhibited its maximum stability at pH 11. This result suggested that the protease produced belonged to the class of alkaline protease. The effect of different temperatures was studied to find out the temperature suitable for the activity and stability of the protease. The result showed greater activity at 60°C. Evaluations of the agro-industrial wastes indicated that corn husk and chicken feathers resulted in the maximum production of the protease in all the other optimum conditions.

The industrial demand of proteases with novel and better properties continues to stimulate the researchers in this area. For the production of proteases for industrial use, isolation, purification and characterization of new promising strain are continuous processes. Although different alkaline proteases have been isolated from several bacteria and fungi, few have better properties that can be commercially exploited.

References

Abdullah F.M. 2006. The production of extracellular protease using Bacillus subtilis: effect of temperature and agitation speed. BSc Thesis. *University College of Engineering and Technology. Malaysia.* 46p.

Aruna K, Shah J, Birmole R. 2014.Production and partial characterization of alkaline protease from Bacillus tequilensis strains CSGAB0139 isolated from spoilt cottage cheese. *Int J Appl Biol Pharma Tech*: 5: 201-221.

Asha, B., &Palaniswamy, M. 2018. Optimization of alkaline protease production by Bacillus cereus FT 1 isolated from soil, 8(02), 119–127.

Badhe P, Joshi M, Adivarekar R. 2016. Optimized production of extra cellular proteases by Bacillus subtilis from degraded abattoir waste. *J Bio Sci Biotechnol:* 5: 29-36.

Bajaj BK, Jamwal G.2003.Thermostable alkaline protease production from Bacillus pumilus D-6 by using agro-residues as substrates. Adv Enzyme Res: 1:30-36.

Banerjee UC, Sani RK, Azmi W, Soni R.1999. Thermostable alkaline protease from Bacillus brevis and its characterization as a laundry detergent additive. *Proc. Biochem*. 35: 213-219.

Boominadhan U, Rajkumar R, Sivakumaar PKV, Joe MM. 2009. Optimization of protease enzyme production using Bacillus Sp. isolated from different wastes. *Bot Res Int*: 2:83-87.

Brammacharry, U. 2010. Production and characterization of protease enzyme from *Bacillus laterosporus*.

Dorcas K, Pindi PK. 2016. Optimization of protease production from Bacillus cereus. *Int J Curr Microbiol Appl Sci:* 5:470-478.

Deng, A., Wu, J., Zhang, Y., Zhang, G., & Wen, T. 2010. Bioresource Technology Purification and characterization of a surfactant-stable high-alkaline protease from Bacillus B001. *Bioresource Technology*, 101(18), 7100–7106.

El Zawahry YA, Awny M, Tohamy EY, AbouZeid AAM, Reda FM. 2007. Optimization, characterization and purification of protease production by some Actinomycetes isolated under stress conditions. *Proceeding of The Second Scientific Environmental Conffer, Zagazig Uni*: 153-175.

Faranak, S., Oskouie, G., Tabandeh, F., Yakhchali, B., & Eftekhar, F.2008. Response surface optimization of medium composition for alkaline protease production by *Bacillus clausii*, 39, 37–42.

Frankena J., Koningstein G.M., van Verseveld H.W., Stouthamer, A.H. 1986, Effect of different limitations in chemostat cultures on growth and production of exocellular protease by Bacillus licheniformis. *Appl Microbiol Biotechnol*; 24:106–12.

Gençkal, H. 2004. Studies on Alkaline Protease Production from Bacillus sp. MSc Thesis. *İzmir Institute of Technology, İzmir, Turkey*. 98p.

Gessesse, A., Hatti-Kaul R., Gashe B.A and Mattiasson B. 2003. Novel alkaline proteases from alkaliphilic bacteria grown on chicken feather. *Enzyme and Microbial Technology*, 32(5): 519-524.

Ghafoor, A., and Hasnain, S. 2009. Production dynamics of Bacillus subtilis strain AG-1 and EAG-2, producing moderately alkaline proteases. *African Journal of Microbiology Research,* 3(5): 258-263.

Gupta A, Khare SK. 2007. Enhanced production and characterization of a solvent stable protease from solvent tolerant *Pseudomonas aeruginosa Pse A. Enzyme Microb Technol,* 2007: 42:11-16.

Gupta, R., Q.K. Beg, S. Khan and B. Chauhan. 2002b. An overview on fermentation, downstream processing and properties of microbial alkaline proteases. *Appl Microbiol Biotechnol.* 60(4): 381-95.

Haddar, A., Agrebi, R., Bougatef, A., Hmidet, N., Sellami-Kamoun, A., and Nasri, M. 2009. Two detergent stable alkaline serine-proteases from Bacillus mojavensis A21: purification, characterization and potential application as a laundry detergent additive. *Bioresource Technology,* 100: 3366-3373.

Hema, T.A and Shiny, M. 2012, Production of Protease Enzyme from Bacillus Clausii Sm3. *IOSR Journal of Pharmacy and Biological Sciences* 1: 37-40Holt, J.G., N.R. Krieg, P.H.A. Sneath and J.T. Staley, 1994. Bergey's Manual of Determinative Bacteriology.

Hoshino E, Maruta K, Wada Y, Mori K. 1995.Hydrolysis of human horny cells by alkaline protease: morphological observation of the process. *J Am Oil Chem Soc*: 72:785-79.

Huang, Q., Y. Peng, X. Li, H. Wang, and Y. Zhang. 2003. Purification and characterization of an extracellular alkaline serine protease with dehairing function from Bacillus pumilus. *Curr. Microbiol.* 46, 169-173.

Ikram. N. 2008. Enhanced production of thermostable bacterial proteases and their applications isolated from natural habitats. *Enzyme Microb. Technol.,* 39, 703-710.

Jayakumar, R., Jayashree, S., Annapurna, B. *et al. Appl Biochem Biotechnol.* 2012. 168: 1849.

Jayasree D, Sandhya Kumari TD, Kavi Kishor PB, Vijayalakshmi M, Lakshmi Narasu M. 2009.Optimization of production protocol of alkaline protease by Streptomyces pulvereceus. *Inter JRI Sci Technol*: 1(2):7982.

Joo, H., & Chang, C.2005. Production of protease from a new alkalophilicBacillus sp . I-312 grown on soybean meal : optimization and some properties, 40, 1263–1270.

Kalpana Devi, M., RasheedhaBanu, A., Gnanaprabhai, G.R., Pradeep, B.V., and Palaniswamy, M. 2008. Purification, characterization of alkaline protease enzyme from native isolate Aspergillusniger and its compatibility with commercial detergents. *Indian Journal of Science and Technology,* 2008; 1:16.

Kalwasinska, A., Jankiewicz, U., Felfoldi, T., &Burkowska-but, A.2018. Alkaline and Halophilic Protease Production by Bacillus luteus H11 and Its Potential Industrial Applications.

Khusro A. 2015. Statistical approach for optimization of independent variables on alkali-thermo stable protease production from Bacillus licheniformis strain BIHPUR 0104. *Electron J Biol*: 11:93-97.

Kumar CG, Tiwari MP, Jany KD. 1999. Novel alkaline serine proteases from alkalophilicBacillus spp: Purification and some properties. Proc. Biochem. 34: 441-449.

Lakshmi, B. K. M., Sri, P. V. R., Devi, K. A., & Hemalatha, K. P. J. 2014. Original Research Article Media optimization of protease production by Bacillus licheniformis and partial characterization of Alkaline protease, 3(5), 650–659.

Mabrouk, S.S., Hashem, A.M., El-Shayeb, N.M.A., Ismail, A.M.S., and AbdelFattah, A.F. 1999. Optimization of alkaline protease productivity by Bacillus licheniformis ATCC 21415. *Bioresource Technology*, 69 (2): 155159.

Marathe, S.K., Vashistht, M.A., Prashanth, A., Parveen, N., Chakraborty, S., and Nair, S.S. 2018. Isolation, partial purification, biochemical characterization and detergent compatibility of alkaline protease produced by Bacillus subtilis, Alcaligenesfaecalis and Pseudomonas aeruginosa obtained from sea water samples. *Journal of Genetic Engineering and Biotechnology*, 16(1): 39-46.

Maurer, K.2004. Detergent proteases, 330–334.

Nadeem, M. 2009. Biotechnological production of alkaline protease for industrial use. PhD Thesis. *University of Punjab, Lahore, Pakistan*. 208p.

Olajuyigbe FM, Ehiosun KI. 2013. Production of thermostable and organic solvent-tolerant alkaline protease from Bacillus coagulans PSB-07 under different submerged fermentation conditions. *Afr J Biotechnol*: 12:3341-3350.

Pant, G., Prakash, A., Pavani, J.V.P., Bera, S., Deviram, G.V.N.S., Kumar, A., Panchpuri, M., and Prasuna, R.G. 2015. Production, optimization and partial purification of protease from Bacillus subtilis. *Journal of Taibah University Science*, 9: 50-55.

Pastor MD, Lorda GS, Balatti A. 2001.Proteases obtention using Bacillus subtilis- 3411 and amaranth seed meal medium at different aeration rate. *Braz J Microbiol*: 32(1):6-9.

Rahman, R.N.Z.A., Geok, L.P., Basri, M., and Salleh, A.B. 2005. Physical factors affecting the production of organic solvent tolerant protease by Pseudomonas aeruginosa strain K. *Bioresource Technology*, 96(4): 429436.

Rathod, M.G., and Pathak, A.P. 2016. Optimized production, characterization and application of alkaline proteases from taxonomically assessed microbial isolates from Lonar soda lake, India. *Biocatalysis and Agricultural Biotechnology*, 7: 164-173.

Ray, A. 2012. Protease Enzyme- Potential Industrial Scope Review: *Int. J. Tech.* 2(1): 01-04.Research 3(3): 653-669.

Sánchez-Porro, C., Mellado, E., Bertoldo, C. *et al.* 2003. *Extremophiles*. 7: 221.

Saraswathy N, Yeole GS, Parikh AJ, Meena C. 2013. Production and optimization of protease from Bacillus licheniformis NCIM 2044. *Asian J Pharma Life Sci:* 3:9-15.

Selim S, Hagagy N, Aziz MA, El-Meleigy S., Pessione E. 2014. Thermostable alkaline halophilic-protease production by *Natronolimnobiusinnermongolicus* WN18. Nat Prod Res: 28:1476–9.

Sen, S. and Satyanarayana, T.1993.Optimization of alkaline protease production by thermophilic Bacillus licheniformis S-40. *Indian Journal of Microbiology*. 31:43-47.

Sevinc, N. and E. Demirkan. 2011. Production of Protease by Bacillus sp. N-40 Isolated from Soil and Its Enzymatic Properties. *J. Biol. Environ. Sci.*, 5(14), 95-103.

Sharma, K.M., Kumar, R., Vats, S., Gupta, A. 2014. Production, partial purification and characterization of alkaline protease from *Bacillus aryabhattai* K3. *International Journal of Advances in Pharmacy, Biology and Chemistry*, 3(2): 290-298.

Shumi W, Hossain MT, Anwar MN.2004.Proteolytic activity of a bacterial isolate Bacillus fastidious den Dooren de Jong. *J Biol Sci*: 4:370-374.

Singhal, P., V. K. Nigam and A.S. Vidyarthi. 2012. Studies on production, characterization and application of microbial alkaline proteases.

Sumantha, A., C. Larroche and A. Pandey. 2006. Microbiology and Industrial Biotechnology of Food-Grade Proteases: A Perspective. Food Technol. Biotechnol. 44 (2) 211–220.

Tambekar S D, Tambekar D H. 2013. Optimization of the production and partial characterization of an extracellular alkaline protease from thermo-halo-alkalophiliclonar lake bacteria. Biosci Discov: 4:30-38.

Vanitha N, Rajan S, Murugesan AG.2014. Optimization and production of alkaline protease enzyme from Bacillus subtilis 168 isolated from food industry waste. *Int J Cur Micro biol Appl Sci*: 3:36-44.

Vidyasagar M, Prakash S, Mahajan V, Shouche YS, Sreeramulu K.2009. Purification and characterization of an extreme halothermophilic protease from a halophilic bacterium Chromohalobacter sp. TVSP101. *Braz J Microbiol*: 40:12–9.

Votruba, J., Pazlarova, M., Dvorakova. M., Vachova, L., Strnadova, M., Kucerova, H., Vinter, V., Zourabian, R., and Chaloupka, J.1991. External factors involved in the regulation of synthesis of an extracellular proteinase in Bacillus megaterium: effect of temperature. *Applied Microbiology and Biotechnology*, 35(3): 352-357.

Wang, H.Y., Liu, D.M., Liu, Y., Cheng, C.F., Ma, Q.Y., Huang, Q., and Zhang, Y.Z. 2007. Screening and mutagenesis of a novel Bacillus pumilus strain producing alkaline protease for dehairing. Letters in applied Microbiology, 44: 1-6.

Ward OP. 1995. Proteolytic enzymes. In M Moo-Young ed. *Comprehensive Biotechnology*. 3:789-818.

Innovations in Biochemical Techniques (2020) : Page no. 104-111
ASTRAL INTERNATIONAL (P) LTD., New Delhi - 110002

Chapter 8

Immobilization-Methods and Applications

Pramod T.

Dept. of Microbiology, The Oxford College of Science, Bangalore, India
Corresponding author: drpramodtaranath@gmail.com

Immobilization can be elucidated as "the physical internment or localization in a determined region of space with retention of its catalytic activity, which can be used repeatedly and continuously" (Tanaka and Kawamoto, 2004). Immobilization of whole cells is now a well accepted method in the field of enzyme technology, scientifically and industrially. Microbial cells in biological process get immobilized either as an artificial process or as natural phenomena.

In natural habitat the attached cells show significant growth, whereas the artificially immobilized cells are allowed restricted growth. The scientific status is documented by an ever increasing number of publications; the industrial breakthrough is demonstrated by the successful performance of several industrial plants (Chibata 1978; Klein and Vorlop (1985). Ever since the initial reports of the successful application of immobilized cells in industrial applications, several research groups all over world have attempted whole-cell immobilization as a viable alternative to conventional microbial fermentations. This has prompted an interest in designing various bioreactors, and various bioreactor configurations have been reported with variable success. The physiological studies of immobilized cells and development of measuring techniques has enhanced the knowledge on the microbial metabolism under the immobilized state (Ramakrishna and Prakasham, 1999).

Immobilization is an appropriate term covering methods of generation of heterogeneous biocatalysts. In case of enzymes this usually refers to the formation of insoluble complexes, but however in case of cells which are already insoluble, it is mainly related to their deployment within a bioreactor in such a way that they are retained, resulting in a cell free product. The application of immobilized cells as industrial catalysts has various operational advantages associated with the use of immobilized enzymes together with number of additional advantages. Downstream processing for the extraction of intracellular enzymes and their purification often in low yields is not needed. Immobilization of whole cells is inclined to improve the stability of enzymes by retaining them in their natural surroundings during immobilization and their subsequent continuous operation. There are few substantiation to indicate that bound cell systems are more tolerant to the changes in the physical environment like temperature and pH when compared to the immobilized enzymes. The immobilized cells are more tolerant to the toxic substances in the substrate in the form of heavy metals and oxygen, thereby reducing the pretreatment of substrates before scale-up (up-streaming) into the bioreactor. (Venkatasubramanian and Vieth, 1979 and D'Souza, 1989).

Bioprocess industry is significantly influenced by enzyme and microbial technology in recent years by improvement of existing processes as well as in the development of novel eco-friendly industrial processes. Immobilization of cells and enzymes is one of the techniques, which has played a significant role. Immobilization has helped in the retention of the biomass in a reactor geometry thereby enabling their economic reuse and in the development of continuous processes.

Immobilization has helped in improving the stability and preventing contamination problems in bioprocessing. Thus the protection rendered to the cells by immobilization has helped in introducing them into soils for agricultural and environmental applications. Immobilization has also played a important role in the construction of biosensors in establishing contact of the biomaterial on transducer surface and in the field of medicine for the formation of immuno-barrier (D'Souza, 2002).

Currently the immobilized cells are gaining importance as a source of immobilized enzymes. Immobilization of whole cells either can be in a viable or non-viable form. One important limitation in the utilization of whole cells as an intracellular source of enzymes is the diffusion of substrate and products through the cell membrane. One of the ways of finding a solution to the problem is by using permeabilized cells, by using physical and chemical (organic solvents/detergents) techniques. One of the most common techniques is using of organic solvents such as toluene, chloroform, ethanol and butanol or detergents like N-cetyl-N, N, N-trimethyl ammonium bromide (CTAB), sodium deoxycholate and digitonin (D'Souza, 1989, 1999 a,b; Patil and D'Souza, 1997).

Immobilized viable cells are gaining significance in fermentation (D'Souza, 1989; 1999 a,b; Ramakrishna and Prakasham, 1999). One of the challenges for the future biotechnologists is in improving the fermentation techniques. Classical fermentation suffers from various limitations such as low density, nutritional limitations and batch mode of operation with high down times. It is recognized that microbial cell density is of prime importance for attaining higher productivity.

The major problem in the development of continuous fermentation process has been the wash out of cells from the bioreactor.

The use of membrane reactors, flocculating strains and cell recycle are being investigated to find a solution to these problems. Determination of the cell density prior to fermentation is one of the advantages. This facilitates operation of fermentation on a continuous mode without cell washout even at higher dilution rates. In addition to microbial cells the fermentation technology using bioreactors is also gaining importance in the production of high value compounds using plant and animal cell cultures (D'Souza, 2002).

Advantages of Immobilized Cells over Immobilized Enzymes

1. Reduces enzyme purification and extraction steps.
2. Increased yields of enzyme activity after immobilization.
3. Generally higher operational stability.
4. Effectively reduced enzyme cost.
5. Cofactor regeneration.
6. Increased potential for multistep processes.
7. Considerable resistance to environmental changes.

Immobilization Methods

There are a large number of techniques which are now available for the immobilization of cells on different supports. The choice of immobilization technique depends on the nature of the cell, nature of the chemical conversion and its ultimate application in proper reactor geometry. More considerate methods are required often for the immobilization of viable cells compared to the non viable cell systems (D'Souza, 1989).

There are four different types of immobilization methods that can be distinguished. These include entrapment, covalent binding, cross-linking and adsorption.

There is no single system which is applicable to all enzymes or cells as it depends upon the differences in their composition and overall charge distribution. Substrate characteristics also influence the choice of the method of immobilization.

Entrapment of Cells

This is the most frequently used method for immobilizing whole cell systems. This immobilization method does not depend significantly on the cellular properties. The principle of entrapment is to form a polymeric network around the material to be trapped. The gel must have sufficient porosity to allow the transport of substrates in and products out while retaining the cells. Though this technique has minimum constraints on the cells, some charges having localized effects are likely to be introduced by the matrix material (Mosbach, 1976; Messing, 1975; Goldman *et al.*, 1971 and D'Souza, 1989). The cells are free within their compartment and also allow post immobilization growth with simultaneous entrapment, while retaining full viability with possible increase in active biomass within the gel matrix promoting and thus intensifying the process (D'Souza, 1989).

Various natural polymers like alginates, carrageenan, cellulose, agar, agarose, hen egg white, gelatin, collagen, and synthetic polymers like polyacrylamide and other acrylic polymers, photo cross-linkable resins *etc* have been employed for the entrapment of whole cell systems (Tampion and Tampion, 1987 and D'Souza, 1989). Alginate has been extensively investigated for the preparation of immobilized viable cell systems, whereas acrylamide polymerized using either chemical or radiation has shown potential for obtaining immobilized nonviable cell systems (D'Souza, 1989).

Covalent Binding

In this technique of covalent binding the creation of permanent chemical bonds has been extensively used in the immobilization of enzymes. The mechanism involves the covalent bond formation between activated inorganic support and cell in the presence of a binding agent. Covalent binding of enzyme or cell to a solid matrix has the advantage of an attachment which is not reversed by pH or ionic strength. Because of several disadvantages only few systems using this technique have been reported. One of the general issues with covalent binding is that cells are exposed to potent reactive groups, which might exert toxic effects, affecting the viability of the cells.

The covalent binding is applicable to the immobilization of any cell. The surface of the cells contain various reactive groups such as hydroxyl, aldehyde, ketone, carboxyl, amino, sulphydryl, imidazole and other substituted aromatic rings. Thus there is great potential for the creation of covalent bonds with suitable carriers by using the techniques of immobilization. Some of the commonly used coupling agents are gluteraldehyde, carbodiimide, isocyanate and aminosilane (D'Souza, 1989).

Adsorption of Cells

Adsorption of cells is a reversible process. This means that the support may be recovered after the catalyst is denatured. Immobilization of cells through adsorption on solid surfaces is probably the mildest of cell immobilization techniques. It is the cheapest and the simplest method so it is particularly used in the industrial processes of value added products. Adhesion of cells is a natural phenomenon, whereby the organisms adhere to one-another and play an important role in many natural processes. This is the technique normally used in the 'fixed film' or 'trickling filters' and also in the 'fermentation of vinegar'. Adsorption of cells is mainly dependent upon the composition of the carrier, surface-charge, surface area and pore size are some factors that are important in adsorption of cells. Adsorption is also dependent upon the cell wall composition, age, volume and surface area of the cell more importantly the charge they carry, *i.e.* in physiological pH conditions the cells carry a net negative charge. This property is made use in choosing the ion exchangers. The cell wall of Saccharomyces cerevisiae and Candida utilis are composed of a-mannans. Hence these cells can be immobilized on glass surface which is used as a model support bearing a negative charge by coating the cells to be immobilized as a monolayer. Yeasts and bacteria have also been immobilized by passive adsorption on a variety of supports including woodchips, cotton cloth, sawdust, porous bricks, glass and ceramics (D'Souza, 1989).

Cross-linking

Microbial enzymes and cells can be immobilized by cross-linking with bi-functional reagents such as glutaraldehyde, cyanuric chloride, *etc.* Among these glutaraldehyde has been extensively used in view of its GRAS status (Mattiasson,

1983; Tampion and Tampion, 1987). Cross-linking itself may find little practical application because of the formation of only fine insoluble precipitates which may not be possible for use in bioreactor systems; the production is also low due to the inactivation by extensive cross-linking. Recently, techniques have been developed for the adsorption followed by cross-linking with glutaraldehyde which is being used for the immobilization of certain enzymes. Cells have been normally immobilized in the presence of an inert protein like hen egg white, gelatin and collagen using glutaraldehyde as cross-linker. This technique has advantages and disadvantages of both entrapment and cross-linking. This technique has been commercially used in the production of high fructose syrups (D'Souza, 1989; Ramakrishna and Prakasham, 1999).

Application of Immobilized Cells

Antibiotic Production by Immobilized Microbial Cells

One of the key areas in the field of applied microbiology is antibiotic production. Conventionally it is produced in stirred tank batch reactors, as it is a non growth associated process. It is difficult to produce the antibiotic in continuous fermentation with free cells, hence immobilization of cells has been found to be suitable since growth and metabolic production can be controlled without affecting the metabolite yields. Several attempts have been made for the production of antibiotics wherein the cells of Penicillium chrysogenum has been immobilized for the production of Penicillin G. These cells were immobilized in k-carrageenan and used for the batch and continuous production of penicillin and compared with the cells immobilized on celite, in which they observed that the immobilized cells on celite were more productive than the cells immobilized on k-carrageenan. Reports suggest that immobilized cells were better producers than the free cells (Ramakrishna and Prakasham, 1999). Mahmoud and Rehm (1987) in their studies entrapped Penicillium chrysogenum in calcium alginate and used them in bubble column reactors with limited success. Reports on the studies on antibiotics is also available on the production of Bacitracin, Patulin, Nikkomycin, Neomycin, Candidicin, Cephalosporin, Erythromycin, Actinomycin D and Cyclosporin (Ramkrishna and Prakasham 1999)

Enzyme Production

Microorganisms are the best sources for the production of commercially important enzymes. Whole cell immobilization technology is aptly suited for the production of extracellular enzymes. There is a growing interest in applying cell immobilization techniques for the continuous production of enzymes. Among the enzymes, Extensive studies have been carried out on the degradation of starch by α-amylases and glucoamylases. Several workers have attempted the production of these enzymes through the immobilization of cells. Entrapment of cells in polyacrylamide, calcium alginate, agar and several other polymer supports have been attempted. Ramakrishna and Prakasham, 1999 reported the immobilization of Bacillus cereus in calcium alginate and employed packed bed and fluidized bed reactors for the continuous production of thermostable α-amylases. There are also reports on the production of thermophilic α -amylase from transformed cells of E. coli immobilized in k-carrageenan with supplementation of glycine. Among various supports/matrices attempted silicone foam was reported to be the best for the entrapment of *E. coli* EC 147 for the production of α-amylases. Similarly A. niger strains were immobilized by some workers for the production of glucoamylases. Among the various matrices tried for the immobilization, k-carrageenan and alginate were the most effective (Ramakrishna and Prakasham, 1999).

Fiedurek and Szczodrak attempted the passive immobilization of A. niger by physical adsorption on wheat, whey, barley and mustard seeds. Mycelium grown on the mustard seeds exhibited highest enzyme activity and can be repeatedly used. Several studies on the immobilization of *Trichoderma reesei* for the production of cellulases from cellulosic materials have been investigated. The immobilizations of these fungi on polyester cloth, non-woven material and cellulosic fabric have been attempted. In recent years the immobilization of various microbial cells namely Rhizopus chinens

A. niger, Candida rugosa and *Sporotrichum thermophile apinis* for the production of lipases has been attempted. Immobilization of *Phanerochaete chrysosporium* for the production of lignin peroxidases has been a subject of great interest and the immobilization of this fungi are reported by several workers (Ramakrishna and Prakasham, 1999). In addition to the above enzymes several other enzymes like proteases, α-galactosidases, xylanases, invertases have also been produced by immobilized cells.

Production of Alcohols

Immobilized cells of yeast are one of the widely studied systems for ethanol fermentation. Almost all the immobilization methods, namely gel entrapment, adsorption on various carriers, cross-linking were tried for alcohol fermentation. There are reports on the immobilization of *Zymomonas mobilis* for alcohol production. Many reactors are being operated on a continuous basis with better results. The immobilization of yeast on ceramic like matrix material of aluminium silicate composition has been reported. There are also reports on the immobilization of *Zymomonas mobilis* in polyurethane for the higher production of alcohol. Nojima reported the large scale continuous alcohol fermentation by immobilized cells of yeasts. The yeast cells were mixed with photo- cross linkable resin and were polymerized by light sources. There are reports on the immobilization of S. *cereviceae* using calcium alginate as matrix for the production of alcohol.

Organic Acid Production

Organic acids are important microbial products which find their application in food and medicines. Amongst the various organic acids, citric acid holds predominant position as a commercial biochemical. The widely used microorganism for the synthesis of citric acid is *Aspergillus niger.* In the conventional batch fermentation *A. niger* is employed for citric acid production. The serious disadvantage in the fungal fermentations is the increasing viscosity during growth, which lead to poor oxygen supply to the cells, thereby necessitating the supply of the sterile air. In such cases the immobilization of cells play an important role wherein the growth of the cells is restricted and the operation of the fermentors becomes simple. The most widely used methods for the immobilization of *A. niger* cells are the entrapment in alginate gels, agarose and polyacrylamide. In addition adsorption on various supports, such as polyurethane foam and entrapment in hollow fibres has been attempted. Fuji *et al.*, tried porous cellulose carrier as support matrix for *A. niger* and observed that the immobilized cells enhanced the productivity substantially. Khare *et al.* (1994) successfully utilized soy whey as substrate than the conventionally used sucrose as substrate.

There are a few reports on the use of yeast *Yarrowia lipolytica,* in immobilized phase for the production of citric acid. Kautola *et al.* (1991) have evaluated several carriers such as alginate, k-carrageenan, polyurethane gel, nylon web, and polyurethane foam for active and passive immobilization of the cells. Among all these the cells entrapped in alginate have shown highest citric acid productivity. It has been observed that the immobilized cells of *A. niger* require low initial sucrose concentration than the free cells for maximum productivity. High sucrose concentrations led to reduced yield and high polyol formation.

Immobilization of cells has also been used for the fermentative production of lactic acid. *Lactobacillus helveticus, L. delbrueckii, L. casei, Rhizopus oryzae* and *Pedioccus halophilus* are the important microorganisms used for the production of lactic acid by immobilized cells. Since there are many reports on the shrinkage of the alginate beads during lactic acid fermentation, Audet *et al.*, 1988 reported a method of immobilization of cells in a mixture of k-carrageenan and locust bean gum, which showed significant stability for 3 months in continuous fermentation in stirred tank reactors.

Several workers have reported the fungal fermentation of acetic acid by the cells of *Acetobacter* sps. immobilized in hollow fibres, ceramic supports and carrageenan. Some workers have also reported the production of acetic acid using the alginate immobilized beads of *Acetobacter aceti* cells. Various other organic acids produced by immobilization such as itaconic acid, malic acid, propionic acid, gluconic acid, fumaric acid, gibberlic acid succinic acid and butryic acid have also been reported (Ramakrishna and Prakasham, 1999).

References

Audet, P., Paquin, C. and Lacroix, C., Appl. Microbiol. Biotechnol., 1988, 29, 11–18.

Chibata, I., in Enzyme Engineering (ed. Brown, G. B.). Plenum Press, New York, Vol. 4. 1978.

D'Souza S.F. 1989b Potentials of co-immobilizates in biochemical processing: The current state of the *Art. J. Microbial Biotechnology* 4:63-73.

D'Souza S.F. 1999b. Immobilized cells in biochemical process development and monitoring in the advances in bioprocessing and r DNA Technology ed. V.Bihari and S.C. Agarwal, Modern Printers, Lucknow, India,pp107-125

D'Souza S.F.1989a Immobilized Cells: Techniques and applications. Ind. J. of Microbiology, 29:83-117.

D'Souza S.F.1999a Immobilized enzymes in bioprocess. Curr. Sci. 77:69-79.

D'Souza, S.F. and Kubal B. S. 2002 Cloth strip bioreactor containing immobilized glucoamylase. *J. Biochem. Biophys. Methods* (in press)

Goldman, R., Goldstein, L., and Katchalski, E, (1971) In Biochemical Aspects of Reactions on Solid Supports, G. R. Stark, ed., p. 1, Academic Press, New York, New York.

Kautola, H., Rymowicz, W., Linko, Y-Y. and Linko, P., Appl. Microbiol. Biotechnol., 1991, 35, 447–449.

Khare S.K., Vaidya S., and Gupta, M.N. 1991,Entrapment of proteins by aggregation within sephadex beads Appl. Biochem. Biotechnol. 27(3): 205-16.

Klein and Vorlop 1985, Immobilization Techniques-Cells. In: Comprehensive Biotechnology2, New York.

Mahmoud, A. H., El Sayed, M. and Rehm, H. J., Appl. Microbiol. Biotechnol., 1987, 26, 215–218.

Mattiasson, B. 1983. Immobilized Cells and Organelles. CRC Press, Boca Raton, FL.

Messing R. A. (Ed). 1975, Immobilized engineering for industrial reactions. Academic Press, New York.

Patil and D'Souza S.F. 1997, Measurement of insitu halophilic glyceraldehydes 3 phosphate dehydrogenase activity from the permeabilized cells of Archaebacterium Haloarcula valismortis. J. *Gen. Appl. Microbiol.* 43:163-167.

Tampion. J and Tampion,M.D. 1987, Immobilized Cells: Principles and Application. Cambridge University Press, Cambridge UK.

Venkatasubramanian K, Vieth WR 1979, Immobilized microbial cells. In: Bull MJ (ed). Progress in Industrial Microbiology, 15. Elsevier, Amsterdam, Oxford, New York, pp 61–86.

Innovations in Biochemical Techniques (2020) : Page no. 112-124
ASTRAL INTERNATIONAL (P) LTD., New Delhi - 110002

Chapter 9

Nanotechnology: Current uses and Future Applications in Agri and Food Sector

P. Sreevani

Head of the Department of Botany, Dr.V.S.Krishna Govt. Degree & PG College (A), Visakhapatnam, Andhra Pradesh. Ph:9908369522, Email: srvani6@gmail.com

Abstract

The field of nanotechnology is one of the most popular areas for current research and development in basically all technical disciplines. Recent advances in nanoscience and nanotechnology intend new and innovative applications in the Agriculture food industry. Nanotechnology exposed to be an efficient method in many fields, particularly the Agriculture and food industry. Agri-food themes focus on sustainability and protection of agriculturally produced foods, including crops for human consumption and animal feeding. Nanotechnology provides new agrochemical agents and new delivery mechanisms to improve crop yield and productivity, and it promises to reduce pesticide use. Nanotechnology can boost agricultural production, and its applications like nanoformulations of agrochemicals for applying pesticides and fertilizers for crop improvement, the application of nanobiosensors in crop protection for the identification of diseases and residues of agrochemicals, nanodevices for the genetic manipulation of plants, plant disease diagnostics, animal health, animal breeding, poultry production and postharvest management. Precision farming techniques could be used to further improve crop yields but not damage soil and water, reduce nitrogen loss due to leaching and emissions, as well as enhance nutrients long-term incorporation by soil microorganisms. Raising awareness of nanotechnology in the agri-food sector, including feed and food ingredients, intelligent packaging and quick-detection systems, is one of the keys to influencing consumer acceptance. This review highlights the applications of current nanotechnology research in food technology and agriculture, including nanoemulsion, nanocomposites, nanosensors, nano-encapsulation, food packaging, and propose future developments in the developing field of agrifood nanotechnology.

Keywords: *Agriculture, food sector, nano science, yield and productivity, agro chemicals*

Introduction

Nanotechnology can contribute to the development of innovative applications in the agriculture, food and feed sector (hereinafter referred to as agri/feed/food) with new and enhanced properties (Chaudhry, Q. *et al* 2008). Applications include nano-encapsulated agrochemicals or nutrients, antimicrobial nanoparticles and active and intelligent food packaging. It is expected that applications will increase in the future and thereby represent a relevant source of direct exposure of humans to nanomaterials. The use of nanomaterials in food is a highly contentious topic, and many people are diametrically opposed to the concept of consuming foodstuffs "tainted" by nanotechnology. Nanotechnology has the potential to revolutionize the global food and agricultural system. Nanoscale control of food molecules could allow the modification of many macroscale characteristics of foods, such as texture, sensory attributes, processability, and shelf life. The tools of nanotechnology have already allowed scientists to better understand the way in which food components are structured and how they interact with each other. This understanding is expected to enable a more precise manipulation of food molecules for the design of healthier, tastier, and safer foods.

Global food industry is under rising pressure to meet consumers demand for safe, healthy and fresh food, along with a challenge to meet updated strict food safety regulations. Awareness through easy access to digital media have motivated consumer toward demand for fresh, minimally processed, nutritious, safe and ready-to-eat food products with well-defined labels. In-order to make certain the safety and authenticity of food stuffs throughout the food supply chain, food manufacturers, traders, buyers and food regulatory authorities seeks a novel, cost-effective, fast and consistent tool to monitor the packaged food quality; more effectively to the traditional passive barrier concept, as packaging is a crucial component of every segment of food industry (Janjarasskul and Suppakul, 2016; Sarkar *et al.*, 2017). Nano-technological interventions to food packaging chiefly explore three possibilities viz. direct incorporation into food products, incorporation in food packaging material, and application in food processing. The commercialization, successful execution and responses to diverse applications of nanotechnology are determined by the consumer's outlook toward and acceptance of newly introduced technologies and their applications (Gupta *et al.*, 2011; Kim *et al.*, 2014). Outcome from majority of the studies (apart from those of sample population) indicates wide consumer acceptance of nanoparticles as packaging materials and also when they are used during processing activities; as compared to their direct incorporation into agri-food products (Giles *et al.*, 2015).

The concept of nanotechnology was introduced in 1959 by Richard Feynman and the term "nanotechnology" was later coined by Norio Taniguchi in 1974. Nanotechnology mainly comprises of fabrication, characterization and manipulation of nano-range (<100 nm) molecules. The application of nanotechnology in polymers involve the design, manufacturing, processing and application of polymer materials filled with nano-particles and/or devices of nano range (Paul and Robeson, 2018; Danie *et al.*, 2013; Momin and Joshi, 2015). The enormous potential of this promising intervention has gained attention of researchers from multi-disciplinary areas *i.e.,* biological sciences, chemistry, engineering and physics. Owing to high global interest, nanotechnology has been proposed to impact the global economy by around $3 trillion by 2020, generating a requirement of approximately 6 million professionals in different inter-related sectors (Duncan, 2011). As predicted by the Institute for Health and Consumer Protection (IHPC), the nanoparticle based market will touch $20 billion mark by 2020 (Belli, 2012; Montazer and Harifi, 2017). It can be anticipated that nanotechnology will create a major thrust for the development of advanced packaging systems for the sake of consumers. Differently from the materials at macroscale, nanomaterials display specific and improved physicochemical properties. By virtue of their small size, nanoparticles hold a huge surface-to-volume ratio and surface activity. When affixed to desirable polymers, nanomaterials results in improved mechanical strength, electrical conductivity and thermal stability *etc.* Nanomaterials thus improve the mechanical and barrier properties of food packages; along with offering active and intelligent packaging systems (Mihindukulasuriya and Lim, 2014). The rapid development of nanotechnology has been facilitating the transformations of traditional food and agriculture sectors, particularly the invention of smart and active packing, nanosensors, nanopesticides and nanofertilizers. Numerous novel nanomaterials have been developed for improving food quality and safety, crop growth, and monitoring environmental conditions. In this review the most recent trends in nanotechnology are discussed and the most challenging tasks and promising opportunities in the food and agriculture sectors from selected recent studies are addressed. The toxicological fundamentals and risk assessment of nanomaterials in these new food and agriculture products are also discussed. We highlighted the potential application of bio-synthesized and bio-inspired nanomaterial for sustainable development. However, fundamental questions with regard to high performance, low toxic nanomaterials need to be addressed to fuel active development and application of nanotechnology. Regulation and legislation are also paramount to regulating the manufacturing, processing, application, as well as disposal of nanomaterials. Efforts are still needed to strengthen public awareness and acceptance of the novel nano-enabled food and agriculture products. We conclude that nanotechnology offers a plethora of opportunities, by providing a novel and sustainable alternative in the food and agriculture sectors.

Some of the benefits of nanotechnology will be conveyed to the food system directly through agriculture and agricultural research. Newly created tools in molecular and cellular biology will enable significant advances in reproductive science and technology, disease prevention, and treatment of plants and animals and potentially boost the production of raw food materials. The development of biosensors for pathogen and contaminant detection in agricultural products will help ensure the safety of the food supply. Conversion of renewable agricultural materials or food waste into energy and useful by-products is an environmentally oriented area of research that could be greatly enhanced by nanotechnology. The heated debates surrounding this issue are not without precedent. Similar discussions about the use of genetically modified (GM) foods were extremely common all over the world and effectively triggered the demise of the industry before it had the opportunity to take off—despite broad scientific consensus that GM food poses no greater risk to health than does conventional food. However, in the case of GM foods, However, rather than nanomaterials that occur through traditional fabrication methods, the real controversial issues appear to center on the addition of artificial nanomaterials and the use of nanotechnology to engineer beneficial properties in foodstuffs (Kah, M. *et al.* 2013). Apparently the use of nanomaterials as a means of advancing food technology is currently at a crossroads similar to the one that GM food faced in the 1990s, and many factors including potential benefits, potential risks, Nutritive value and public perception stand to play an important role in determining the eventual chances of success for what could one day become a multi-billion-dollar industry.

Nanotechnology and Food for Animals

Nanotechnology involves manipulation of materials on an atomic or molecular scale. It is an emerging technology that has the potential to be used across the spectrum of FDA-regulated products, including animal food. FDA has not established regulatory definitions of "nanotechnology," "nanomaterial," "nanoscale," or other related terms. In June 2014, FDA issued a guidance for industry entitled, "Considering Whether an FDA-Regulated Product Involves the Application of Nanotechnology." As described in that guidance, at this time, when considering whether an FDA-regulated product involves the application of nanotechnology, FDA will ask: (1) whether a material or end product is engineered to have at least one external dimension, or an internal or surface structure, in the nanoscale range (approximately 1 nm to 100 nm) and (2) whether a material or end product is engineered to exhibit properties or phenomena, including physical or chemical properties or biological effects, that are attributable to its dimension(s), even if these dimensions fall outside the nanoscale range, up to one micrometer (1,000 nm) (Aschberger. K et. al. 2014)

Nanotechnology and Food Safety

One of the new technologies to improve food safety is nanotechnology, which is the manipulation or self-assembly of individual atoms, molecules, or molecular clusters into structures, the purpose of which is to create materials and devices with new or vastly different properties. Nanotechnology will enable the manufacture of high-quality products at a very low cost and fast pace. It is commonly referred to as a generic technology that offers better-built, safer, longer-lasting, cheaper, and smarter nonfood products with wide applications in consumer households, the communications industry, and the medicine field. For food manufacturers, using nanotechnology can mean gaining a more competitive position. While in the long term consumers may benefit from advances in nanotechnology as new methods for improving the safety and quality of food products are developed and applied, the products still need to be regulated to ensure safety and consumer protection.

Current and Future Applications of Nanotechnology in Agri/Feed/Food

Most of the records in the Nano Inventory concern applications in food (almost 90%) with food additives and food contact materials being the most frequent types of application. A much smaller percentage of applications in the Nano Inventory is concerned with agriculture (9%) and feed (3%). 55 different types of NM, both inorganic and organic, can be found in the Nano Inventory. The most frequent types of NM are nano-encapsulates, silver and titanium dioxide.

Applications of NM in agriculture include improved and targeted pest management and crop protection through increased efficacy, durability, bioavailability and controlled release of pesticides and other agrochemicals (Kah, M. and T. Hofmann 2014). This can for example be achieved by nano-encapsulation or binding active substances to solid lipid nanoparticles or porous solid particles (*e.g.* silica) (Frederiksen, H.K 2003 ; Liu, F. *et al.* 2006). Nanotechnology can also enhance crop production and thereby potentially reduce the quantity of fertiliser that has to be applied (Kole, C. *et al.* 2013). Nanotechnology is also applied for detection of animal and plant pathogens, and for identity preservation and tracing and the slow release of nutrients or active compounds used in veterinary drugs (Underwood, C. and A.W. van Eps 2012 ; Parisi C. V.M., Rodríguez-Cerezo E 2014). Food nanotechnology has infiltrated into many aspects of customer products, such as food packaging, additives, and food preservation. The recognition of this novel technology has advanced the food processing and storage in ensuring food safety. Many conventional chemicals added as food additives or packaging materials have also been found partially existing at nanometer scale. For example, food-grade TiO2 NPs now have been found up to approximately 40% in the nanometer range Dorier et. al.2017 ; Dudefoi et. al. 2017. Although nanomaterials like TiO2 NPs are generally recognized low toxic at ambient conditions, long term exposure to such nanomaterials may cause adverse damages Weir. A *et. al.* 2012. The application of novel food nanotechnology, together with the presence of nanoscale chemicals, has also attracted public attention regarding the potential risks.

Nanomaterials in Items of Food

Potentially, nanoscale additives to food could bring a raft of benefits. Other potential applications include the encapsulation of vitamins and mineral supplements that would boost the health benefits of consuming certain foods without having a detrimental effect on taste or nanoscale salt crystals that, as a result of the higher surface area, would give the same taste from significantly lower volumes of overall material enabling people to cut down their overall salt intake. Some commentators also suggest that nanotechnology could aid in the battle against food shortages particularly in the developing world. An additional 2 billion mouths to feed by 2050 means that novel food-production methods will be necessary to avert a potential global crisis.

Despite the potential benefits that nanotechnology could bring to the food industry, very few nanomaterials currently find use in food products. Although not strictly a foodstuff, one product that can contain a variety of nanoscale additives is toothpaste. Nanoparticles of hydroxyapatite a naturally occurring substance in teeth and bones coat teeth and fill in cracks. The particles break down when in contact with acidic fluids and thus sacrificially protect the enamel in teeth from attack (Chaudhry, Q. *et al.* 2008). The additive is also a source of calcium and phosphate ions that can aid in the remineralization of the surface of teeth. Some manufacturers also add silver nanoparticles a well-known antibacterial agent to toothpastes, reducing gum disease and, in turn, bad breath. In sufficiently high concentrations, silver nanoparticles can, however, be highly toxic, and as a result of tight regulations their use in toothpaste is not common outside Asia. Nano and microscale particles of titanium dioxide a strong white pigment also find use in some toothpastes. The use of titanium dioxide nanoparticles in foodstuffs is particularly controversial because the nanonparticles offer no real benefits other than color enhancement. Titanium dioxide nanoparticles can accumulate in the small intestine, and although medical practitioners are currently unaware of any adverse health ramifications, the use of nanoparticles in foodstuffs for purely cosmetic reasons is questionable and may not justify the potential risk.

Although nanotechnology is not currently widely in use in the food industry, other routes by which humans can ingest nanoscale materials remain. Nanomaterials are increasingly gaining regulatory approval for use in medical applications. Efficient cancer therapies as well as a variety of novel drug-delivery techniques are just two applications that nanomaterials are currently enabling. These measures, which by necessity must undergo rigorous regulatory procedures, could potentially open the door to more general applications that may be of interest to the food industry (Kah, M. and T. Hofmann 2014). The potential also exists for human ingestion of nanomaterials through the food chain by, for example, the administration of antibiotics to animals or the use of pesticides or fertilizers on crops. Strict regulations must be in place to avoid any potentially harmful or unwanted ingestion of nanomaterials through these routes.

Nanomaterials in Food Packaging

Food packaging is one area in which nanotechnology is already making a significant impact in the food industry. Potential applications of advanced or "smart" packaging range from the advanced for example, the introduction of packaging that keeps food fresh for longer than does standard packaging or that incorporates sensors that inform users whether the items inside are still fresh to the less radical for instance, the use of stronger, lightweight composites that enable an overall reduction of material necessary to package items of food.

The application of nanoparticles is explored in numerous sectors such as electronics, medicine, textiles, defense, food, agriculture, and cosmetics. Nanotechnology caters several areas of food sciences such as food safety, packaging, processing, bioavailability, fortification, encapsulation, pathogen detection *etc.* (Weiss *et al.*,2006; Ravichandran, 2010). Nanotechnology based food packaging offer numerous advantages over conventional food packaging materials via improving several properties such as temperature resistance, enhanced durability, flame resistance, barrier, recycling and optical properties, processability due to lower viscosity; proficiently delivery of active materials into the biological systems, at minimum costs with lessen environmental issue. Such progressions make it an ideal candidature for the development of nano materials in wide array of food packaging applications such as processed meat and meat products, cheese, confectionery, cereals, boil-in-the-bag foods, in addition to this it also helps in extrusion-coating applications for fruit juices and dairy products, or co-extrusion processes for the manufacture of bottles for beer and carbonated drinks (Bumbudsanpharoke and Ko, 2015; Trujillo *et al.*, 2016).

In general, nanoclay-plastic composites are up to 100 times stronger than regular plastics, which means that less material is necessary in the packaging of food. In addition, nanoclay, when embedded into polylactic acid a biodegradable plastic that finds use in food packaging causes the material to degrade at a faster rate than do standard biodegradable plastics, helping to regulate a substantial environmental problem.

Materials such as copper and silver nanoparticles can function as antibacterial agents in food packaging and help inhibit the spread of harmful microbes. However, metallic nanoparticles can also aid in keeping food specifically fruit fresh by acting as a catalyst that breaks down ethene gas that ripening fruit produces and that also accelerates the ripening process. The removal of ethene from warehouses that store perishable items is an extremely important commercial process, with previous. attempts at using biotechnological methods proving prohibitively expensive or ineffective (Dekkers, S. *et al.* 2011)

Safety concerns, although less pronounced than in the case of nanoscale food additives, persist with food packaging. Most scientific studies conclude that the risk of human exposure through the migration of nanoparticles from packaging to food is minimal. However, public-health bodies tend to promote a cautionary approach. Human exposure is not the only concern. The risks of environmental contamination remain high, and legislators must take into account these risks alongside any perceived benefits when considering approval for the widespread use of these materials. Nanotechnology-enabled food packaging currently finds use in the most of the developing countries.

Toxicological Data and Risk Assessment

The main focus of pharmacology and toxicology is the desired and undesired or adverse effects of chemical substances on living organisms. One important task in this field is the identification of the basic mechanisms of action that means, the interaction between the chemical substance and the biological structures relevant for the effect at the molecular level. Understanding the toxicological effects of substances thus requires sound knowledge of physiology and biochemistry to answer the question about the mode of action of a poison or drug.

The often described people's lack of understanding pharmacology and toxicology is probably mainly caused by the general non-existence of the necessary basic knowledge. Both pharmacological and toxicological facts are often poorly understood. For instance, the development and use of immunosuppressive agents is a key requirement of transplantation medicine. Yet, the ordinary person seems to comprehend surgical interventions better than the mode of action of immune suppressants which requires at least basic knowledge of the function of the immune system. As a consequence, medical advances in this field become more commonly associated with surgery than with pharmacology and are not viewed as interdisciplinary research success. Data and information stored in the Nano Inventory indicate that silica, silver and titanium dioxide are the most common NM in toxicity testing and risk assessment. The most tested toxicity end points include genotoxicity, acute toxicity, cytotoxicity and repeated dose toxicity. Very often the physicochemical characterisation of the NM is very poor and was reported in less than 15% of the records concerning (eco)toxicity and risk assessment of NM.

Biological Natural Nano Particles

Biological naturally occurring nanoparticles (nanoclay, tomato carotenoid lycopene, many chemicals derived from soil organic matter, lipoproteins, exosomes, magnetosomes, viruses, ferritin) have diverse structures with wide-ranging biological roles. Biological nanoparticles are often biocompatible and have reproducible structure. Potential biomedical applications of natural and modified biological nanoparticles have been reported (Stanley.S 2014).

Animals use nanotechnology, where nanostructures help animals climb, slither, camouflage, flirt, and thrive. A good example is the ordered hexagonal packed array of structures in the wings of cicadas (for instance, Psaltoda claripennis Ashton) and termites (for example, family Rhinotermitidae) Zhang.G et.al.2006). Studying nanostructured nipple arrays of moth eye facets helps to design better thin-film solar cells (Dewan.R et.al. 2012). A combination of three functions in one biological nanostructure (antiadhesive properties of insect ommatidia grating in addition to their widely accepted antireflective properties and ability to reduce glare to predators) can be exploited for the development of industrial multifunctional surfaces capable of enhancing light harvesting while reducing light reflection and adhesion (Peisker and Grob 2010). Butterfly wings contain nanostructures that give rise to optical effects such as iridescence, the effect of changing color when viewed from different angles (Tam et.al. 2013). The tokay gecko uses nanotechnology to stick itself to trees, walls, windows, and even ceilings. Mimicking the agile gecko, researchers have created synthetic "gecko tape" with four times the sticking power of the real thing (Science dialy 2007). It is well known that insects possess ferromagnetic resonance which is temperature dependent and that magnetic nanoparticles in social insects act as geomagnetic sensors (Esquivel. D.M.S. 2007).

Nanotechnology promises to improve current agriculture practices through the enhancement of management and conservation of inputs in crops, animal production, and fisheries (Thornton.P.K. 2010). In recent years, the food industry has made great progress in areas such as the improvement of new packaging products, the development of new functional products, transport and controlled release of bioactive substances, detecting of pathogens by using nanosensors and indicators, and purification of water through the use of nanoparticles (Senturk. A., et.al. 2013 ; Boom 2011). The potential for improving the effectiveness of agricultural active ingredients using nanosized particles, including functionalized nanocapsules, has been reported. (Zhao *et. al.* 2012). Agricultural applications also include i) nanotechnology-enabled delivery of agriculture chemicals, ii) field-sensing systems to monitor the environmental stresses and crop conditions, and iii) improvement of plant traits against environmental stress and diseases.(Forsberg E.M. et. al. 2013 ; Scott N.R. 2014 ; Joseph. T. et.al. 2006 ; Owolade O.F. et.al. 2008 ; Knauer. K. and Bucheli. T.D. 2009 ; Manimegala. G et. al. 2011)

Conclusion

Nanotechnology applications in the agricultural, feed and food sector are growing and novel products are expected to enter the market in the near future. An up-to-date knowledge on the occurrence and type of application of NM in this sector is vital to estimate the potential human exposure to NM from food and feed. It is also becoming increasingly important that the regulatory frameworks properly address and specifically manage the potential risks of nanotechnology. Several countries over the world have been particularly active in examining the appropriateness of their regulatory frameworks for dealing with nanotechnologies but have applied different approaches to address safety issues of nano-based products in agri/feed/food: from legally binding provisions to guidance for industry.

Despite massive potential benefits, use of nanomaterials in the traditionally conservative food industry remains limited to a handful of applications. A key factor that will determine the extent to which if at all nanotechnology will affect the food industry is public perception of safety and risk. The general public will likely have difficulty in accepting "unnatural" nanoscale food additives unless compelling and risk-free health benefits exist. Regulatory challenges also pose a large barrier to rapid development within the sector. All Open dialogue between scientists, key industrial players, and consumers must exist in order to overcome any negative perceptions and enable nanotechnology to fulfill its potential in the food industry.

he quality of food items chiefly rely over their perishability. Perishable foods require ambient temperature to maintain quality and freshness during transit and storage. Monitoring the extent to which perishable foods encounter degradation promoting factors chiefly, oxygen, light and ethylene can control perishability. Food package and the packaging material involved play an important and decisive role in food quality and shelf life. Packaging chiefly influences the barrier properties to form an irrefutable food environment. The dawn of nanotechnology has further opened up new avenues and technological advancement possibilities in food packaging area. Linking of nanoparticles to polymer to fabricate nanomaterial packaging potentiates routine packaging with enhanced barrier properties, mechanical and thermal strength, flexibility and stability. Time-consuming quality-control analysis as well as consumer technical illiteracy is another key problem surfacing the food industry. Novel nano-packaging systems (Improved/Active/Intelligent packaging) have potential to serve as an important tool to overcome existing packaging challenges with consumer and industrialist satisfaction. It is anticipated that conventional packaging will be thoroughly replaced with multifunctional smart or active packaging. Nano-structured materials put a check to microbial invasion, assuring microbial food safety. Additionally, nanosensors alert and warn consumers regarding the safety and accurate nutritional status of the packaged food. Several corporations have entered in this area with introduction of new packaging systems with updated technology. However, being a young branch, gaps in knowledge exists, leaving ample questions to the scientific community; mainly concerning its toxicity and ecotoxicity. Concerns regarding nanoparticles migration to packaged foodstuffs has been raised, however, migration assays and risk assessment are still not conclusive. Undefined toxicity, scarcity of supportive clinical trials data and risk assessment studies limits the application of nanomaterial in the food packaging sector.

References

Aschberger K, S Gottardo, V Amenta, M Arena, F Botelho Moniz, H Bouwmeester, P Brandhoff, A Mech, L Quiros Pesudo, H Rauscher, R Schoonjans, M Vittoria Vettori and R Peters. (2014). Nanomaterials in Food - Current and Future Applications and Regulatory Aspects. *Journal of Physics. Conference Series, Volume* 617.

Belli B. (2012). Eating Nano: Processed Foods and Food Packaging Already Contain Nanoparticles - Some of Which Could be Harmful to Our Health. The Environmental Magazine.

Boom RM. Nanotechnology in food production. In: Frewer LJ, Norde W, Fischer ARH, Kampers FWH, editors. Nanotechnology in the Agri-Food Sector: Implications for the Future. Weinheim, Germany: Wiley-VCH; 2011. pp. 39–58.

Bumbudsanpharoke N., Ko S. (2015). Nano-food packaging: an overview of market, migration research, and safety regulations. *J. Food Sci.* 80, R910–R923. 10.1111/1750-3841.12861

Chaudhry, Q., *et al.*, Applications and implications of nanotechnologies for the food sector. Food Additives and Contaminants - Part A Chemistry, Analysis, Control, Exposure and Risk Assessment, 2008. 25(3): p. 241-258.

Chaudhry, Q., L. Castle, and R. Watkins, Nanotechnologies in Food. RSC Nanoscience & Nanotechnology. Vol. 25. 2010, Cambridge: Royal Society of Chemistry. 229.

Dekkers, S., *et al.*, Presence and risks of nanosilica in food products. Nanotoxicology, 2011. 5(3): p. 393-405.

Danie K. J., Shivendu R., Nandita D., Proud S. (2013). Nanotechnology for tissue engineering: need, techniques and applications. *J. Pharm. Res.* 6, 200–204. 10.1016/j.jopr.2013.02.021

Dorier M., . Béal, D Marie-Desvergne C., Dubosson M.,. Barreau, F, . Houdeau. E, *et al.* Continuous in vitro exposure of intestinal epithelial cells to E171 food additive causes oxidative stress, inducing oxidation of DNA bases but no endoplasmic reticulum stress Nanotoxicology, 11 (2017), pp. 751-761

Dudefoi.W, Terrisse. H., Richard-Plouet, E. Gautron, F. Popa, B. Humbert, *et al.*

Criteria to define a more relevant reference sample of titanium dioxide in the context of food: a multiscale approach Food Addit Contam A, 34 (2017), pp. 653-665

Dewan R, Fischer S, Meyer-Rochow VB, Özdemir Y, Hamraz S, Knipp D. Studying nanostructured nipple arrays of moth eye facets helps to design better thin film solar cells. *Bioinspir Biomim.* 2012;7(1):016003.

Giles E. L., Kuznesof S., Clark B., Hubbard C., Frewer L. J. (2015). Consumer acceptance of and willingness to pay for food nanotechnology: a systematic review. *J. Nanopart Res.* 17:467. 10.1007/s11051-015-3270-4

Gupta N., Fischer A. R. H., Frewer L. J. (2011). Socio-psychological determinants of public acceptance of technologies: a review. *Public Underst. Sci.* 21, 782–795.

Frederiksen, H.K., H.G. Kristensen, and M. Pedersen, Solid lipid microparticle formulations of the pyrethroid gamma-cyhalothrin—incompatibility of the lipid and the pyrethroid and biological properties of the formulations. *Journal of Controlled Release,* 2003. 86(2–3): p. 243-252.

Forsberg EM, de Lauwere C. Integration needs in assessments of nanotechnology in food and agriculture. *Etikk i Praksis.* 2013;1(1):38–54.

Joseph T, Morrison M. Nanoforum Report: Nanotechnology in Agriculture and Food, European Nanotechnology Gateway. 2006. [Accessed April 18, 2014].

Kah, M. and T. Hofmann, Nanopesticide research: Current trends and future priorities. *Environment International,* 2014. 63(0): p. 224-235.

Kah, M., *et al.,* Nanopesticides: State of Knowledge, Environmental Fate, and Exposure Modeling. *Critical Reviews in Environmental Science and Technology,* 2013. 43(16): p. 1823- 1867.

Kim Y. R., Lee E. J., Park S. H., Kwon H. J., An S. S., Song S. W., *et al.* (2014). Comparative analysis of nanotechnology awareness in consumers and experts in South Korea. *Int. J. Nanomedicine* 15, 21–27.

Kole, C., *et al.,* Nanobiotechnology can boost crop production and quality: first evidence from increased plant biomass, fruit yield and phytomedicine content in bitter melon (Momordica charantia). *BMC Biotechnology,* 2013. 13(1): p. 37.

Knauer K, Bucheli TD. Nano-materials: research needs in agriculture. Revue Suisse d'Agriculture. 2009;41(6):337–341.

Liu, F., *et al.,* Porous hollow silica nanoparticles as controlled delivery system for watersoluble pesticide. *Materials Research Bulletin,* 2006. 41(12): p. 2268-2275.

Manimegalai G, Kumar SS, Sharma C. Pesticide mineralization in water using silver nanoparticules. *International Journal of Chemical Sciences.* 2011;9(3):1463–1471.

Momin J. K., Joshi B. H. (2015). Nanotechnology in foods, in Nanotechnologies in

Food and Agriculture, eds Rai M., Ribeiro C., Mattoso L., Duran N., editors. (Springer International Publishing;), 3–24.

Montazer M., Harifi T. (2017). New approaches and future aspects of antibacterial food packaging: from nanoparticles coating to nanofibers and nanocomposites, with foresight to address the regulatory uncertainty, in Food Package, ed *Grumezescu* A. M., editor. (Academic Press;), 533–559.

Owolade OF, Ogunleti DO, Adenekan MO. Titanium dioxide affects diseases, development and yield of edible cowpea. EJEAFChe. 2008;7(5):2942–2947.

Parisi C., V.M., Rodríguez-Cerezo E., Proceedings of a workshop on "Nanotechnology for the agricultural sector: from research to the field"in JRC Scientific and Policy Report 2014, Publications Office of the European Union, 2014: Luxembourg.

Paul D. R., Robeson L. M. (2008). Polymer nanotechnology: nanocomposites. Polymer 49, 3187–3204. 10.1016/j.polymer.2008.04.017.

Ravichandran R. (2010). Nanotechnology applications in food and food processing: innovative green approaches, opportunities and uncertainties for global market. *Int. J. Green Nanotechnol. Biomed.* 1, P72–P96, 10.1080/19430871003684440.

Peisker H, Gorb SN. Always on the bright side of life: anti-adhesive properties of insect ommatidia grating. *J Exp Biol.* 2010;213(Pt 20):3457–3462.

Sarkar P., Choudhary R., Panigrahi S., Syed I., Sivapratha S., Dhuma C. V. (2017). Nano-inspired systems in food technology and packaging. Environ. Chem. Lett. 10.1007/s10311-017-0649-8

Scott NR. Nanotechnology opportunities in agriculture and food systems; Biological and Environmental Engineering, Cornell University NSF Nanoscale Science and Engineering Grantees Conference; December 5, 2007; Arlington, VA. [Accessed April 19, 2014].

Senturk A, Yalcýn B, Otles S. Nanotechnology as a food perspective. *J Nanomater Mol Nanotechnol.* 2013;2:6.

Stanley S. Biological nanoparticles and their influence on organisms. Curr Opin Biotechnol. 2014;28:69–74.

Tam HL, Cheah KW, Goh DTP, Goh JKL. Iridescence and nano-structure differences in Papilio butterflies. *Optical Materials Express.* 2013;3(8):1087–1092.

Thornton PK. Livestock production: recent trends, future prospects. Phil Trans R Soc B. 2010;365(1554):2853–2867.

Trujillo L. E., Ávalos R., Granda S., Guerra L. S., País-Chanfrau J. M. (2016). Nanotechnology applications for food and bioprocessing industries.

Underwood, C. and A.W. van Eps, Nanomedicine and veterinary science: The reality and the practicality. *The Veterinary Journal*, 2012. 193(1): p. 12-23.

Weir. A. Westerhoff, P. Fabricius, L., Hristovski, K., Von Goetz. N.,Titanium dioxide nanoparticles in food and personal care products. *Environ Sci Technol*, 46 (2012), pp. 2242-2250

Weiss J., Takhistov P., Mc Clements D. J. (2006). Functional materials in food nanotechnology. *J. Food Sci.* 71, R107–R116.

Zhang G, Zhang J, Xie G, Liu Z, Shao H. Cicada wings: a stamp from nature for nanoimprint lithography. *Small.* 2006;2(12):1440–1443.

Zhao M, Liu L, Her R, *et al.* Nano-sized delivery for agricultural chemicals. In: Tiddy G, Tan R, editors. Nano Formulation. Cambridge, UK: Royal Society of Chemistry; 2012. pp. 256–265.

Innovations in Biochemical Techniques (2020) : Page no. 125-137
ASTRAL INTERNATIONAL (P) LTD., New Delhi - 110002

Chapter 10

Current Prominence of Vesicular-Arbuscular Mycorrhizal (VAM) Fungi for Agriculture Crop Investment

Lingayya Hiremath, Ajeet Kumar Srivastava, Narendra Kumar S, Praveen Kumar Gupta and Raksha M.

Department of Biotechnology, RV College of Engineering, Mysore Road, Bangalore–560059, Karnataka, India, lingayah@rvce.edu.in

Abstract

In recent years, there is an increased demand for fertilizers for different reasons like, to prevent pathogen attack on crops, to increase the agricultural yield *etc.* However, this is creating many problems like soil pollution, water pollution, increase in cost of energy *etc.* All these problems can be solved by using a novel organism called Vesicular-Arbuscular Mycorrhizal (VAM) Fungi as a bio fertilizer. During 19th century, discovery of fungal structures colonizing roots led to the initiation of research on arbuscular mycorrhiza. Later, during the second half of the 20th century, research on symbiotic association between plants and fungi was carried in 2 different directions they are cellular and subcellular directions, other is ecology. Symbiotic association between certain phycomycetous fungi and angiosperms or gymnosperms or pteridophytes or bryophytes or also some aquatic roots without causing any harm to the plant is called as Vesicular-Arbuscular (VA) mycorrhiza. It generally has low host specificity. It obtains their nutrients from the plant and provide mineral elements like N, P, K, Ca, S and Zn to the host plant. VAM fungi is responsible to improve growth of host plant species due to increase in nutrient uptake, production of growth promoting substances, tolerance to salinity, alkalinity, toxicities, drought and synergistic interactions with other beneficial microorganism. These fungi play a very important role in decreasing the use of chemical fertilizers in agriculture and simultaneously increase the yield. In this chapter we would discuss in detail about the structure of VAM fungi, mechanism involved by VAM to suppress the soil borne pathogens, the crops which shows positive response to VAM fungi(growth and yield of maize, rice, tomato plant) and also the future research in mycorrhizal technology.

Keywords: *Mycorrhiza, VAM, symbiotic association, ecological interactions, synergistic interactions.*

Introduction

Plants associate with other forms of life (including animals, fungi ,bacteria *etc.*) to complete their life cycle, to thrive in adverse conditions, and also to fight against pathogens. The plant roots and its associated living organisms are collectively called as 'Rhizosphere'. Mycorrhiza is one of the best example for association between plants and fungi. The mutually beneficial relationship that exists between the roots of plants and the fungus that conquers the roots of plants is called as Mycorrhizae. "Fungus-root" is the literal translation of Mycorrhizae. The mutual beneficial relationship between the mycorrhizae and the plants involves, uptake of nutrients and water by plants which is provided by these fungi, and taking shelter and food by fungi which is provided to them by the plants. In nature, more than 80% of angiosperms and almost all gymnosperms are found to have mycorrhizal associations. There are 2 types of mycorrhizal association with plants: Ectomycorrhizae - they may either grow on the surface of the roots (eg. Laccaria bicolor, Amanita mascaria *etc*) and Endomycorrhizae – here the fungus grows inside the plants roots (*e.g.* Endogone, Rhizophagus, *etc.*)

Ectomycorrhizae (EcM)

An ectomycorrhizal is a form of symbiotic association that usually occurs with the woody plants, including birch, oak, spurce, beech, willow, dipterocarp ,and fir. Only about 2% of the terrestrial plant species is found to have ectomycorrhizae. An ectomycorrhiza cannot penetrate into the host cell wall, they form a highly branched hyphae between the epidermal and cortical root cells, which is known as Hartig net. Additionaly, Ectomycorrhizae can be identified by the formation of a thick hyphal sheath which surrounds the root's surface. This is called as mantle. This mantle can be up to 4 µm thick, and the hyphae can extend upto several centimetres. This supports the water and nutrient uptake by plants and also helps the host plant to survive in any adverse circumstances.

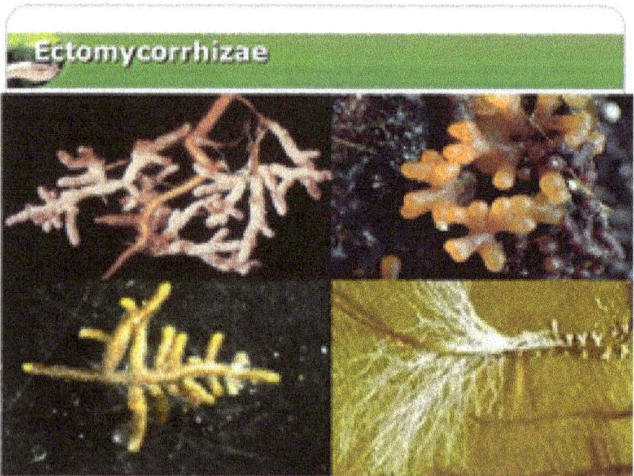

Endomycorrhizae

It is a form of association in which the hyphae of the fungi penetrates and colonizes fleshy cortical cells and epidermal cells of plant roots. About 85% of the plant families in the world is colonized by endomycorrhizae. Endomycorrhizae can occur on most of the seed bearing plants (except those which are colonized by ectomycorrhizae), agricultural crops and enormous variety of the ornamental plants. The association of endomycorrhiza with ornamental plants has paramount application and benefits in ornamental horticulture industry.

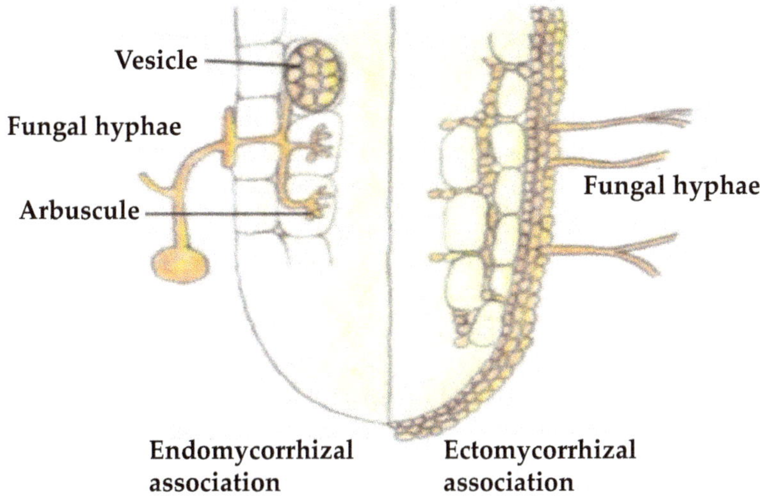

Fig 1: Shows the difference between the endomycorrhizal and ectomycorrhizal association with plants.

Endomycorrhizal Structures

Endomycorrhizae have further been classified into five major groups: arbuscular, ericoid, arbutoid, monotropoid, and orchid mycorrhizae.

Arbuscular Endomycorrhizae : It is the most common type of endomycorrhizae. These are classified based on the structures they produce, which includes vesicles and arbuscules The most common type of endomycorrhizae is arbuscular endomycorrhizae. They are named based on the structures they produce, arbuscules and vesicles.

- **Arbuscules**: They are named by Gallaud (1905). Endomycorrhizae begins to colonize the roots by secreting an enzyme called as arbuscular mycorrhizae. This enzyme allows the hyphae to penetrate into the fleshy cortical cells and the epidermal cells of the plant roots. Arbuscles are formed by repeated reduction in hyphal width dichotomous branching starting from an initial trunk hypha and terminating in a propagation of fine branch hyphae. After 2 to 3 days, the hyphae forms structures within the plant cells called as arbuscles. These arbuscles resemble tiny trees and facilitate the transfer of nutrients within the cortical cells. Hence, they help in delivering certain fertilizer elements and water from soil to plants, and in turn these fungi gets shelter and sugars and other carbohydrates. Arbuscles are short lived and begin to collapse after few days, but hyphae and vesicles can persist in roots for many months or years.

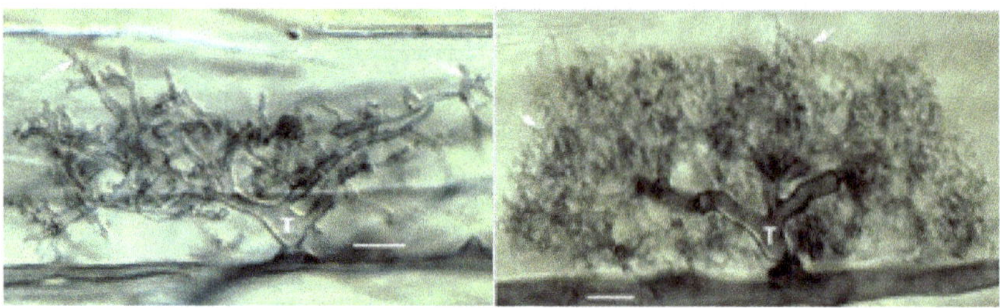

Fig 2(a) **Fig 2(b)**

Fig 2(a): It shows the development of arbusle of Glomus mosseae in the root cell where the arrows shows fine branches and T shows that the arbuscle is branched from an intercellular hyphae.

Fig 2(b): It shows the mature arbuscle of glomus with branches and the main trunk.

- **Spores**: the arbuscular endomycorrhizae hyphae also gives rise to spores. These have the same function as the seeds of plants do. These have thick walls and hence they are highly resistant to intense heat and freezing.
- **Vesicles**: At the terminal ends or midway of hyphae we find the sac like structures called as vesicles. They contain lipids and act as primary storage organs for the fungus. Sometimes vesicles also serve as propagules that can colonize other parts of the plant root.

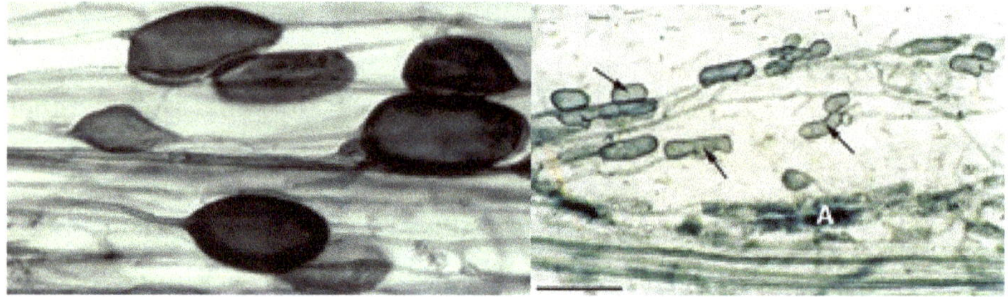

Fig 3(a) **Fig 3(b)**

Fig 3(a): It shows the vesicles produced by Glomus species in leek root.

Fig 3(b): It shows the lobed vesicles of Acaulospora in clover root.

Vesicular – Arbuscular Mycorrhiza (VAM)

Mycorrhizal associations produced by glomeromycotan fungi is known as VAM. But because a main suborder lacks the ability to form vesicles in the roots, AM is usually a preferred acronym. The order Glomales is further divided into many families and genera according to the method used by them for spore formation, structure of their soil borne spores and their DNA sequence.

Table

They are thought to have occupied the similar soil habitats for millions of years, and slowly they have started adapting to changes in the environmental conditions of that particular site. It is formed by the symbiotic association between angiosperm roots and certain phycomycetous fungi. This fungi forms a mycelial network by colonizing the root cortex. This network has characteristic arbuscular(finger like branched structure) and vesicles (bladder- like structures) as discussed above.

Structure and Developmental Stages

1. **Soil hyphae:** This step deals with the initiation step. The initiation may be either by spore germination or due to the fragments of roots. Usually there is a pre-spore germination which has a limited capacity to grow. It will usually die within 1 week if does not encounter any susceptible roots. The hyphae which is emerged due to germination is usually shielded within the spore in Acaulospora and scutellospora species. Figure 5

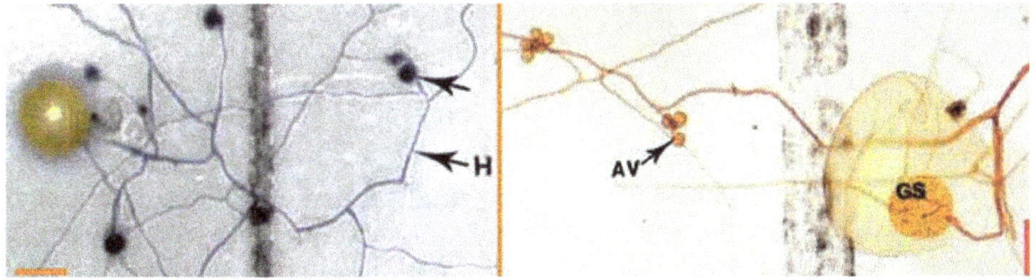

Fig 4: The figure shows the germinated hyphae which is developed from the spores of *Gigaspora decipiens* (left) and *Scutellospora cerradensis* (right).

2. **Root contact and penetration:** Soil hyphae grows towards it as a response of presence of a root nearby the soil hyphae. And hence it institutes a contact with the root and starts to grow along its surface. Now one or more hyphae produces some swellings between the epidermal cells called as appressoria. Later the hyphae penetrates into the cortical or epidermal cells so that they can get access to enter the roots. They enter into the passage cells and cross the hypodermis and start to branch in the outer cortex.

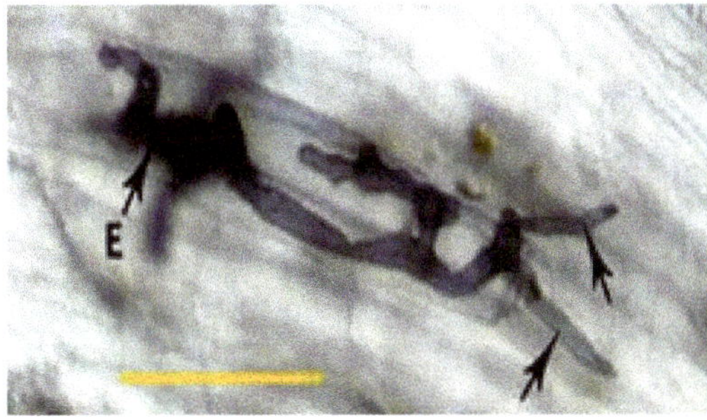

Fig 5: Shows the penetration of the hyphae into the cortex cells of the root. Where 'E' shows the entry point and the 'arrows' shows the penetration point.

3. **Hyphal proliferation in cortex**: Aseptate hyphae extend or spread along the ccortex in both the directions to form a colony. Hyphae which is present within the roots are initially without cross walls, but these might occur in older roots. There are 2 modes of spread within the cortex of roots which are illustrated below:

- **Linear:** These are the type of association where the hyphae of VAM fungi grow longitudinally between the walls of root cells. The consequential colonies have a linear appearance.

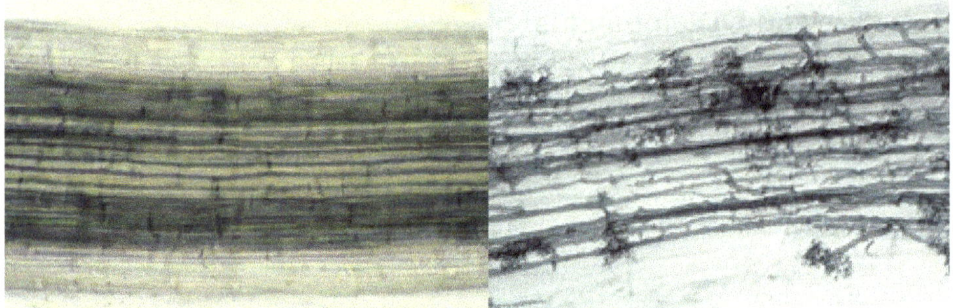

Fig 6: Shows the longitudinal growth of hyphae of VAM fungi on *Allium porrum* (left) and *Glomus versiforme* (right).

- **Coiling:** The colonies of VAM fungi generally have a coiled look. In this type of association the hyphae spread principally by intercellular growth succeeding a convoluted path through the cortex cells. There are various benefits for plants due to the symbiotic association with VAM.

Some of them are listed below

- The symbiotic association of VAM with plants helps in changing the ecology of the given site and hence it helps in mineral recycling and hence helps in increasing the quality of the soil.
- They help in increasing the tolerance of plants against biotic and abiotic stresses which includes toxicity which occurs due to mineral imbalance ,heavy metals and also due to mining operations, alkalinity, soil salinity.
- The VAM fungi can be used as a bio fertilizer and hence it can reduce the use of harmful or chemical fertilizers.
- Produce more vigorous and healthy plants by enhancing flowering and fruiting.
- Reduce disease occurrence and hence increases the yield quality. And hence VAM can be used as a biocontrol agent in modern sustainable agriculture, in terms of various constraints like reducing the damage caused due to various pathogens, cost effectiveness, environmental friendly and also energy savings.

Advantages of Association of Vam with Different Plants

1. Effect of association of VAM on growth of tomato seedling

Tomato (*Lycopersicon esculentum* L.) is considered as a major vegetable crop in many parts of the world. Tomato also has a particular importance as it is a raw material of agricultural industry in addition of it being consumed as a fresh vegetable. It is a major vegetable plant, and is moderately sensitive to salinity. Because of these importance it is necessary to conduct extensive research on growth conditions under reasonable salinity conditions to produce vegetative growth. The influence of salt concentration on plant growth has been studied by conducting various experiments. It has also been reported that the salt concentration reduces the fresh and dry weight of shoots and roots of tomato plants. Due to the combination of osmotic and specific ion effects of Cl and Na when there is increase in salinity over 4000 μg g-1 may result in the reduction of dry weights, leaf area, plant stem, and roots of tomato. VAM fungi widely occur in saline conditions. Hence an experiment was conducted to find the effect of VAM fungi on the growth of tomato plant under saline conditions. To conduct this experiment the tomato seeds were first planted into polythene trays. These trays were sterilized by immersing in 5% sodium hypochlorite, and later is filled with peatmoss. The trays were kept in greenhouse and was irrigated with water without nutrients until cotyledons leaves emerged. Later it was irrigated with water which contained maxifol when the first leaves emerged. Now all these plants are treated with VAM fungi. After the VAM fungi treatment, saline stress treatment commenced after 4 days. 100mM salt concentration is found to be the limit value to create stress on plants, was preferred. Reference plants were the ones which had no saline treatment performed. These reference plants were watered three times a day and the plants which had saline treatment done were treated with water having 100mM salt concentration at regular intervals. After 3 weeks 10 plants were selected randomly and weighed to determine the dry and wet weight of the plants. It was found that VAM fungi treatment increased the weight of fresh stem and root but they did not have any effect on the dry stem and root. It was also found that chlorophyll a, b and total chlorophyll quantities of tomato plants treated with VAM fungi was high when compared to the reference plant, while the carotenoid level was found to be low. It was also found that the tomato plants grown by associating with VAM fungi had high quality growth and it kept the green colour of the plants.

It was also found that the root colonized with VAM fungi is highly branched which increases the number of root tips, surface area, root volume and also length when compared to non colonized plants and also their adventitious roots diameters are larger

2. Effect of association of VAM on onion

Onion is grown as vegetable and spice crop. Onion is known to check the deposition of cholesterol in blood vessels and helps protects against heart diseases which results from blockage of arteries. It is a rich source of vitamin c, protein calcium and phosphorous. Phosphorous is a very essential macro element for plants, but the concentration of phosphorus in soil is very low (from 0.022-0.5%). Hence, phosphorus concentration in plants is usually increased by addition of large amount of chemicals. But the disadvantage of this includes degradation of soil health and hence affects the microbial diversity, loss of organic matter, erosion and also causes health threat for human beings. So for sustainable production of crops an alternative technology which could replace the inoculation of inorganic fertilizers to some extent is the need of this hour. One of the attractive solution for this problem that has been widely studied during the last decade is inoculation of microorganisms like VAM as they have got the ability to supplement phosphorous, nitrogen, zinc, potassium and various other supplements to plants. One of the experiment which was conducted to check the effect of VAM on the growth of onion plant is explained below.

For this experiment 10 plants were randomly selected in such a way that the marginal effect was avoided and some of the data was recorded related to plant height, bulb fresh weight, bulb dry weight, bulb diameter, total soluble solids (TSS), determination of nitrogen, phosphorous and potassium. Now VAM was applied in the root zone at the time of transplantation. All the required cultural practices which includes irrigation, pest and disease control, weeding *etc.* were done uniformly in all the experimental plots.

The data pertaining to the plant height showed that there was an increased growth of onion in terms of plant height due to increase in the absorbing capacity of roots and hence favouring the uptake of water which results in cell expansion responsible for increase in plant height. VAM may increase the uptake of phosphorous, nitrogen and potassium which also results in increasing the plant height due to increase in cellular protein levels, cell division and meristematic activity of plants and also synthesis of photosynthates. The data pertaining to bulb fresh and dry weight showed an increase in bulb dry weight due to increase in the bulb dry weight due to increase in the plant photosynthetic rate which is achieved due to VAM inoculation and hence there is increase in leaf stomatal conductance. Potassium is an activator of various enzymes which is involved in carbohydrate and protein metabolism and it plays an important role in translocation of photosynthates from leaves to bulb which will be utilized in building up the new cells and tissues finally resulting in increase in the bulb fresh and dry weight. The data relating to bulb diameter and yield showed an increase. This may be due to the increase in the availability and the uptake of zinc, potassium, nitrogen, phosphorous *etc.* by onion plant. In addition, root proliferation and the absorbing capacity for water is increased and hence enhancing the food accumulation by the bulbs also contribute to their increase in yield.

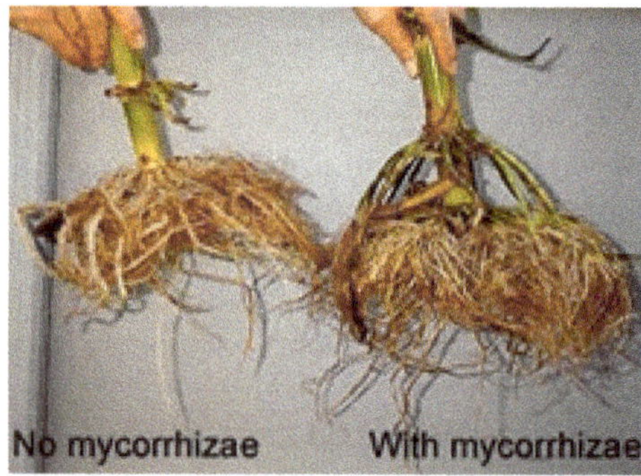

Fig 7: It shows the difference in the onion roots with and without VAM association.

3. Role of VAM on growth and phosphorous nutrition of maize with low soluble phosphate fertilizer:

Some of the soils may be acidic and low fertility. One of the factors that allow the plants to grow on this poor soils is their association with VAM that permits the uptake of immobile phosphorous and other nutrients. VAM fungi also synthesizes and secretes organic substance which are responsible to increase the desoption of phosphorous in liable soil Phosphorous pools. In association with organic acids, VAM fungi can solubilize insoluble and low-soluble phosphorous sources which is a part of minerals (crystalline structures) in soil. This experiment was conducted to investigate and explore the hypothesis which stated that the VAM fungi improved the shoot growth of maize and also the mobilization of phosphorous from low-soluble FePO4. 4H2O. In this experiment the maize was inoculated with spores of VAM fungi. also low-soluble ferrous phosphate was added to the non-mycorrohized and the mycorrohized maize. Now the root of VAM symbiotic plants larger infection when low-soluble phosphorous source was added. It was also found that the shoot and fruit dry weights of non- mycorrhizal maize with added ferrous phosphate was greater than in non-mycorrhizal maize with added ferrous phosphate. This indicates that the non-mycorrhizal plants were able to use the low-soluble phosphorous to only some extent. It was also seen that the dry weight of all mycorrhizal plants was higher than the non-mycorrhizal plants which indicated that VAM fungi enriched the mineral nutrition of maize. To increase the mineral nutrient content ,root length plays a very important role as the length of the root is directly proportional to the nutrient absorbing root surface area. Also the amount of phosphorous in the soil samples from the pots with VAM plants fertilized with P was clearly smaller than that of fertilized non- mycorrohized plants. Also the percentage of phosphorous was higher in the tissues of fertilized mycorrhizal plants. All these results specified that plants in VAM symbiosis mobilize phosphorous efficiently from low-soluble phosphorous when compared to non- mycorrhized plants.

4. Effect of VAM fungi on cucumber at different water regimes

Water availability is known to limit the crop production. Therefore, many researches are going on to study plant water stress interactions both in arid and semi-arid conditions. It is found that VAM fungi that interacts with numerous plants by producing vesicles and arbuscles in root tissue. They are found to have the ability to increase the attainment of ions which are normally slowly diffusing ions through the soil. They are also capable of dissolving weakly soluble minerals present in soil by increasing carbon dioxide partial pressure or releasing acids. Because of all these advantages they enhance the ability of host plants to uptake relatively immobile nutrients predominantly Zn and P. Some studies show that VAM fungi could lessen drought stress in the host plants. When an experiment was conducted on cucumber to find the effect on it due to its association with VAM fungi. The results obtained by this experiment showed that VAM fungi increases the efficiency of the plant water uptake, and results in the gaining greater plant growth. It was found that VAM inoculation increased the total plant yield of fruits receiving about 85% of water regime was considerably higher than that of control plants which received about 100% water regime.

Arbuscular Mycorrhizal Fungi as a Potential Tool in Bio-Control

Plants are always prone to pests. Sometimes the soil borne pathogens were controlled by using various agricultural practices, which includes chemical fungicides, crop rotation, resistant cultivars and soil fumigation *etc.* There are obviously many problems associated with the some of the practices followed *i.e.* over 95% of the herbicides and about 98% of the insecticides sprayed reach a destination other than the target species as they are sprayed across entire agricultural field. Now the runoff can carry the sprayed pesticides into aquatic environment and wind can carry them to other fields, settlements, undeveloped areas and grazing areas finally affecting other species. Other problems may also emerge due to poor transport, production and also storage practices. Because of all these harmful effects, many researchers are trying to use alternate approaches which is based on either adding or manipulating microorganisms to enhance the protection of plants against pathogens. Some of the microorganisms used for biocontrol of pathogens compete with plant pathogens for nutrients and space, by parasitizing pathogens, by producing antibiotics, or by inducing resistance in the host plants. It has also been observed that VAM fungi increases the tolerance of host plant to pathogen attack by compensating for damage in the root biomass by pathogens which may include fungi and nematodes. Some of the soil-borne diseases includes plant pathogenic fungi and root knot disease which is caused by a nematode. All the above mentioned soil-borne disease can be controlled by VAM fungi. Root-knot nematode have been reported to cause yearly loss of up to 23% in egg plant, 22% in okra, 29% in tomato, 28% in beans and so on. These root-knot nematodes and VAM fungi are the members of microbial population near the root region and hence they have the ability to compete with each other for the same site. During this scenario VAM fungi infects nematode and this appears to increase the host tolerance in spite of harming levels of plant parasitic nematode levels. The basis appears to be physiological or physical. VAM fungi helps in increasing the uptake of Ca, Cu, S ,Mn, P and Zn. A plant which is damaged by nematode shows deficiency in uptake of N, B, Mg, Fe, and Zn, it also also impaired water conductance. But VAM fungi induced Zn uptake in plants and also contributing tolerance to Melodogyne incognita in cotton. Hence from the above example it is clear that the VAM fungi can reduce or even eliminate the dangerous effects imposed by root-knot nematodes.

Table 1: Examples for root-knot nematode and VAM fungal interactions studied on varies plants.

Root-Knot Species.	Crop Type	Vam Fungi
M. incognita	Tomato	*Glomus mossaea*
	Papaya	*g. manihotis*
R.citropilus	Citrus	*G.intradices*
R.similis	banana	*G.intradices*
M.hapla	Carrot Onion pyrethrum	*G.mossaea* *G.fasciculatum* *G.etunicatum*
M.javanica and G.mosseae	almond	*G.intradices*

The VAM fungi not only interacts with nematodes but also interacts with microorganisms associated with plants, such as pathogenic fungi. There are almost 10,000 species of fungi which is known to cause disease in plants, and they usually persist in the soil matrix and also resides on soil surface. As discussed earlier the plants infected by VAM high branching rate and also high adventitious root diameter. It was also found that the tomato and cucumber plants colonized by VAM fungi slowed down the infection by Fusarium due to morphological changes in the root cells of these plants which includes lignifications incensement. Hence this rising lignifications may protect the roots from pathogens and also elevating the phenolic metabolism within the host plants. Also when VAM fungi have primary access to the photosynthesis, the greater carbon demand may obstruct the pathogen growth rate.

Table 2: It shows the interaction of various VAM fungi and pathogens in various plants.

Pathogenic fungi	Crops	VAM fungi
S.sinuosa	cotton	G. mosseae
R.solani	alfalfa	G.intradices
M.phaseolina	cowpea	G.fasciculum
A.euteiches	pea	G.intradices

Status and Future Prospects of Mycorrhizal Application

Available summary of publications devoted to the environmental and agricultural benefits of VAM mycorrhiza show their utility in number of crop production. Mainly, wheat, paddy, barley cereals have been investigated with reference to effect of VAM fungi on growth, nutrient uptake and productivity. Attempts have been made to explore the possibility of employing VAM technology in improving the production of vegetables including brinjal, lettuce, potato, onion, tomato, pepper, beans, cucumber and also fruit crops includes papaya, orange, citrus, apple, and banana.

Production of inoculum is expensive due to labor and overhead costs. During research work inoculum is prepared in a very small amount so as to treat a small research plot.

But under field conditions application requires more inoculum. The commercial production of VAM fungi is under process of improvement for past decades. Also with a simple understanding of the biology of VAM fungi and refinement of application techniques for inoculum, the future of environmental conservation and crop improvement using VAM fungi technology seems to be promising.

Conclusion

Worldwide, considerable advancement has been achieved in the area of VAM technology. It has also been validated and proved that VAM fungi have a greater potential for field application so as to improve productivity of vegetables, cereal, fruits and supress nematode and fungal infestations. In terms of efficacy and reliability, the greatest successes in biological control have been achieved by using VAM fungi. Also the public demand to reduce the use of harmful chemicals like pesticides and fertilizers has prompted research on reduction of pesticides and increasing consumer demands for organic food requires the incorporation of VAM fungi.

References

Ahmed A Abdelhafez, Rihan A. Abdel-Monsief.(2006). "Effects of VA Mycorrhizal Inoculation on Growth, Yield and Nutrient Content of Cantaloupe and Cucumber under Different Water Regimes". *Research Journal of Agriculture and Biological Sciences,* 2(6): 503-508.

Al-Karaki GN (2006). Nursery inoculation of tomato with arbuscular mycorrhiazl fungi and subsequent performance under irrigation with saline water. Sci. Hort., 109: 1-7

Akkopru, A. and S. Demir, 2005. Biological control of Fusarium wilt in tomato caused by Fusarium oxysporum f. sp. lycopersici by AMF Glomus intraradices and some rhizobacteria. *J. Phytopathol.,* 153: 544-550.

Dar, Z.M., A. Masood, M. Asif and Malik, M.A. 2018. Response of Onion to Inoculation with Vesicular Arbuscular Mycorrhiza and Phosphorus Solubilizing Bacteria under Varying Levels of Phosphorus. *Int.J.Curr. Microbiol.App.Sci.* 7(02): 2018-2023.

Hakan BAŞAK, Köksal DEMĐR, Rezzan KASIM and F.Yeşim OKAY (2006). The effect of endo-mycorrhiza (VAM) treatment on growth of tomato seedling grown under saline conditions". *African Journal of Agricultural Research Vol.* 6(11), pp. 2532-2538, 4 June, 2011.

Hao, Z., P. Christie, L. Qin, C. Wang and X. Li, 2005. Control of fusarium wilt of cucumber seedlings by inoculation with an arbuscular mycorrhical fungus. *J. Plant Nutr.,* 28: 1961-1974.

J. A. Menge. (1982). Utilization of vesicular-arbuscular mycorrhizal fungi in agriculture. Can. *J. Bot.* 61: 1015-1024.

M. Bansal. K. G. Mukerji (19). Positive correlation between VAM-induced changes in root exudation and mycorrhizosphere mycoflora. *Mycorrhiza* (1994) 5:39-44.

M. H. Dar, Z. A. Reshi, and M. A. Shah(2017). Vesicular arbuscular fungi (VAM) Fungi – as a major biocontrol agent in modern sustainable agricultural system. *Russian Agricultural Sciences,* 2017, Vol. 43, No. 2, pp. 132–137.

Porter, W. M. 1979. The 'most probable number' method for enumerating infective propagules of vesic- ular-arbuscular mycorrhizal fungi in soil. *Aust. J. Soil Res.* 17: 515-519.

Rhodes, L. H., and Gerdemann J. W.. 1975. Phosphate uptake zones of mycorrhizal and nonmycorrhizal onions. New Phytol. 75: 555-561.

Sheng M, Tang M, Chen H, Yang B, Zhang F, Huang Y (2008). Influence of arbuscular mycorrhizae on photosynthesis and water status of maize plants under salt stress. *Mycorrhiza,* 18: 287-296.

Shannon MC, Gronwald JW, Tal M (1987). Effect of salinity on growth and accumulation of organic and inorganic ions in cultivated and wild tomato species. *J. Am. Soc. Hortic. Sci.,* 112: 516-523.

Wang C, Li X, Zhon J, Wang G, Dong Y (2008). Effects of AM fungi on the growth and yield of cucumber plants. *Commun. Soil Sci. Plant Anal.,* 39: 499-509.

Innovations in Biochemical Techniques (2020) : Page no. 138-152
ASTRAL INTERNATIONAL (P) LTD., New Delhi - 110002

Chapter 11

Decolorization of Different Synthetic Dyes by Microorganisms

Vijayakumar Halaburgi

Department of Biochemistry, Gulbarga University, Gulbarga-585106, Karnataka, India.
viji.halaburgi@gmail.com

Abstract

Rapid industrialization, developmental processes or modernization has given rise some unwanted toxic elements into the atmosphere. These elements are accumulated in the biosphere up to toxic level and creating problems in the environment by destroying the natural ecosystem. The textile industry is one of the most polluting industries of clean water. In fact, during the manufacturing processes, a large percentage of the synthetic dye does not bind and is lost in waste waters, which are usually discharged untreated. Textile wastewater is a complex and highly variable mixture of many polluting substances, including dyes, which induce color coupled with organic load leading to disruption of the total ecological balance of the receiving water system. In textile industries 93% of the intake water comes out as colored wastewater due to dyes containing high concentration of organic compounds and heavy metals. The color of wastewater is aesthetically unpleasant to aquatic bodies which hinder the oxygenation ability of water, disturbing the whole of the aquatic ecosystem and food chain. Biological processes by using bacteria, fungi and yeasts are provides alternative technologies that are more cost effective and environmentally friendly.

Keywords: *Bioremediation, Decolorization, Laccase enzyme, Microorganism, Synthetic dyes.*

Introduction

Rapid industrialization has necessitated the manufacture and use of different chemicals in day to day life. The textile industry is one of them which extensively use synthetic chemicals as dyes. Synthetic dyes have increasingly been used in the textile and dyeing industries because of their ease and cost effectiveness in synthesis, firmness, high stability to light, temperature, detergent and microbial attack and variety in color compared with natural dyes. This has resulted in the discharge of highly polluted effluents. Approximately, 10,000 different dyes and pigments are used industrially and over 7×105tons of these dyes are produced annually worldwide (Spadaro *et al.*, 1992).

Textile dyeing effluents containing recalcitrant dyes are polluting waters due to their color and by the formation of toxic or carcinogenic intermediates such as aromatic amines from azo dyes. Water plays a vital and essential role in our ecosystem. This natural resource is becoming scarce, making its availability a major social and economic concern. Use of a large variety of synthetic dyes in textile industries has raised a hazardous environmental alert. About 17-20% of freshwater pollution is caused by textile effluents. The nonbiodegradable nature of the dyes in the spent dye baths of textile industries constitutes a serious environmental hazard. The color of wastewater is aesthetically unpleasant to aquatic bodies which hinder the oxygenation ability of water, disturbing the whole of the aquatic ecosystem and food chain (Xu *et al.*, 2005). These effluents are recalcitrant to biodegradation and cause acute toxicity to the receiving water bodies, as these comprised of various types of toxic dyes, which are difficult to remove. The conventional treatment systems based on physical or chemical treatment does not remove the color and decolorization of textile effluents are very expensive and commercially unattractive (Table 1) (Beydilli *et al.*, 1998).

Microorganisms are able to degrade synthetic dyes to non-coloured compounds or even mineralize them completely under certain environmental conditions. Bioremediation is one of the most effective and successful cleaning techniques for the removal of toxicants from polluted environments (Rodríguez *et al.*, 2006; Singh *et al.*, 2012). The decolorization of the dye takes place either by adsorption on the microbial biomass or biodegradation by the cells and bioremediation takes place by anaerobic and/or aerobic process. Physical and chemical purification methods,including the advanced oxidation processes are not always applicable (Beydilli *et al.*, 1998). They always involve high costs and therefore their use is restricted in scale of operation and pollution profile of the effluent (Robinson *et al.*, 2002). Biological treatment is a more natural wastewater treatment process than other treatment methods(Azmi *et al.*, 1998; Gueu *et al.*, 2007). Microorganisms feed on the complex materials present in the wastewater and turn them into simpler substances, preparing the water for further treatment. Biological methods are currently viewed asspecific, less energy intensive, effective, and environmentally safe since they result in partial or complete bioconversion of organic pollutants to stable and nontoxic end products (Pandey *et al.*,2007; Kumar *et al.*, 2015).

In the present review the decolorization and degradation of synthetic dyes by bacteria and fungi have been cited along with the anaerobic to aerobic treatment processes. The factors affecting decolorization and biodegradation of synthetic dye compounds such as pH, temperature, dye concentration, nitrogen, agitation, effect of dye structure, electron donor and enzymes involved in microbial decolorization of synthetic dyes have been discussed. This paper will have the application for the decolorization and degradation of different synthetic dyes into environmental friendly compounds.

Review of Literature

Many microorganisms belonging to different taxonomic group of bacteria, fungi, actinomycetes and algae have been reported for their ability to decolourize azo dyes and some bacteria are capable to degrade azo, reactive dyes aerobically and anaerobically. This reviews mainly focused on various bacterial and fungal species have been used for decolorization of dyes from the various researchers in their work in world.

Bacterial Methods

Recently number of studies focused the some bacteria are able to biodegrade or bioadsorb the dyes in textile industry effluent (Table 2). The organisms such as Staphylococcus sp, E.coli, Bacillus sp, Clostridium sp. and Pseudomonas sp. were used in most of the dye decolorization study and bacterial decolourization of azo dyes has been reached by sequential anaerobic and aerobic conditions (McMullan *et al.*, 2001; Manjinder *et al.*, 2005). Chen *et al.* (2009) showed the capability of Lactobacillus acidophilus and Lactobacillus fermentum were incubated under anaerobic conditions in the presence of 6 μg/ml Methyl Red, Ponceau BS, Orange G, Amaranth, Orange II, and Direct Blue 15; 5 μg/ml Sudan I and II; or 1.5 μg/ml Sudan III and IV in deMann–Rogosa–Sharpe broth at 37°C for 36 h and both bacteria were capable of degrading all of the water-soluble azo dyes to some extent. Enterococcus faecalis strain YZ66showed complete decolourization of the selected dye (Reactive yellow 145- 50 mg/L) within 10 hours in static anoxic condition at optimum pH 5.0 and temperature 37°C for the decolourization, respectively. Four bacterial isolates (Agrobacterium radiobacter; Bacillus spp.; Sphingomonas paucimobilis, and Aeromonas hydrophila)-(CM-4) were isolated from activated sludge extracted from a wastewater treatment and used to decolorize triphenylmethane dyes. Individual bacterial isolates exhibited a remarkable color-removal capability against crystal violet (50 mg/L) and malachite green (50 mg/L) dyes within 24 h and the microbial consortium CM-4 shows a high decolorization 91% and 99% within 2 hfor crystal violet and malachite green, respectively. UV-Visible absorption spectra, FTIR analysis and the inspection of bacterial cells growth indicated that color removal by the CM-4 was due to biodegradation. Evaluation of mutagenicity by using Salmonella typhimurium test strains, TA98 and TA100 studies revealed that the degradation of crystal violet and malachite green by CM-4 did not lead to mutagenic products (Cheriaa *et al.*, 2012).Plants and bacterial consortium of Portulaca grandiflora and Pseudomonas putida showed complete decolorization of a sulfonated diazo dye Direct Red 5B within 72 h, while in vitro cultures of P. grandiflora and P. putida independently showed 92 and 81% decolorization within 96 h, respectively. Plant and bacterial enzymes in the consortium gave an enhanced decolorization of Direct Red 5B synergistically. The metabolites formed after dye degradation analyzed by UV–Vis spectroscopy, Fourier transformed infrared spectroscopy and High performance liquid chromatography confirmed the biotransformation of Direct Red 5B (Khandare *et al.*, 2013). Galactomyces geotrichum MTCC 1360 exhibited

86% decolorization of azo dye Reactive Yellow-84A (50mgL(-1)) within 30h at 30°C and pH 7.0 under static condition. Considerable reduction of COD (73%) and TOC (62%) during degradation of the dye was indicative of conversion of complex dye into simple products. In addition, when G. geotrichum was applied to decolorize textile effluent, it showed 85% of true color removal (ADMI removal) within 72h, along with a significant reduction in TOC and COD. Phytotoxicity studies revealed the less toxic nature of degraded Reactive Yellow-84A as compared to original dye (Govindwar *et al.*, 2014).The Kerstersia sp. decolourized aerobically seven different naphthalene-containing sulfonated azo dyes such as Amaranth, Fast Red E, Ponceau S, Congo Red, Orange II, Acid Red 151 and Acid Orange 12 at optimum temperature 400C and pH 7.0. The bacterium decolourized Amaranth, Fast Red E, Congo Red and Ponceau S by 100% (100 mg/L) and the remaining three dyes Orange II, Acid Orange 12 and Acid Red 151 were decolourized by 84%, 73% and 44%, respectively in 24 h. About1g/L concentration of Amaranth and Ponceau S were decolourized within 24 h, whereas only 0.6 g/L of Fast Red E was decolourized in 24 h. On the other hand a mixture of all the three dyes at 1 g/L concentration was decolourized within 26 h. The decolourization kinetics of the dyes with azoreductase enzyme supports the ping-pong mechanism.

The Amaranth dye degraded products were extracted and characterized by TLC, diazotization and Carbylamines test, which indicated that Amaranth was biotransformed into non-toxic aromatic metabolite without amine group (Vijayakumar *et al.*, 2007).The Shewanella sp. strain KMK6 was isolated from the dyecontaminated soil and was applied to mixture of dyesunder suitable conditions. The results indicated that the decrease in COD (Chemical Oxygen Demand) and color of the dye mixture with the production of nontoxic degraded products (Kolekar *et al.*, 2013). Decolorization of mixture of dyes and actual textile effluent was done with a novel bacterium Lysinibacillus sp. RGS about 87% decolorization was obtained for mixture of dyes with69% COD reduction after 48 hours (Saratale *et al.*,2013). Under in vitro conditions G. pulchella and P. monteilii showed decolorization of the dye Scarlet RR (SRR) by 97 and 84%, within 72 and 96 h respectively, while their consortium showed 100% decolorization of the dye within 48 h. In case of dye mixture G. pulchella, P. monteilii and consortium-PG showed an ADMI removal of 78, 67 and 92% respectively within 96 h(Kabra *et al.*, 2013). Aeromonas hydrophila a bacterial strain was identified best for color removal at optimum pH 5.5-10.0 and temperature 20-30°C (Naik and Singh, 2012) and Jayan *et al.* (2011) has analysed the decoloration and physico-chemical parameters ofdye mixtureby using Bacillus, a type of bacteria which proved to be efficient in color and COD removal. An ecofriendly strain Brevibacillus laterosporus MTCC 2298 decolorizes mixture containing seven commercial textile dyes with different structures and color properties. It showed 87% effective decolorization of dye mixture in terms of ADMI removal (American Dye Manufacturing Institute) within 24hwas attained in the presence of metal salt-CaCl2, nitrogen sources and phytotoxicity study revealed the much less toxic nature of the metabolites produced after the degradation of dyes mixture (Kurade *et al.*, 2011).Among all tested microorganisms, isolated Sphingobacterium sp. ATM effectively decolorized (100%) the dye Direct Blue GLL (DBGLL) and simultaneously it produced (64%) polyhydroxyhexadecanoic acid (PHD). The organism decolorized DBGLL at 300 mg/Lconcentration within 24 h of dye addition and gave optimum production of PHD. The organism also decolorized three combinations (1. fives days, 2. seven dyes 3. ten dyes) of mixture of dyes having 0.5 g/L concentration and also decolorizes textile effluent when it was combined with medium. The organism produced a maximum of 66% and 61% PHD while decolorizing mixture of dyes and textile effluent respectively and there was significant reduction in chemical oxygen demand (COD) and biological oxygen demand (BOD). The biotransformation of DBGLLFTIR was confirmed by analysis of samples before and after decolorization at optimum temperature 37°C and the rate of decolorization decreased with the increase intemperature (Tamboli *et al.*, 2010). Newly isolated halophilic and halotolerant bacteria (Asad *et al.*, 2007) from coconut coir sample worked efficiently for removal of dyes from mixture. Some newly isolated strains from sludge samples and mud lakes also could efficiently decolorize the mixture of dyes. The strain Shewanella putrefaciens CN32 was firstly applied to decolorize water insoluble Sudan dyes under anaerobic condition at optimum temperature 26°C, pH 7.0-8.0 and NaCl concentrations 0-20 g/L. The decolorization also enhanced by using biosurfactant rhamnolipid and the highest decolorization of 90.23% to Sudan I was achieved within 108 h. The co-culture of S. putrefaciens CN32 and Bacillus circulans BWL1061 is reported for the first time to accelerate the decolorization through improving the synergistic effect of enzymatic degradation and biological reductive effect and the microbial toxicity tests indicated that the toxicity of Sudan I to Escherichia coli BL21 and Bacillus subtilis 168 was obviously decreased after the decolorization, suggesting that co-culture technique has a good potential in the treatment of dyeing wastewater (Liu *et al.*, 2018).

Fungal Methods

A wide variety of fungal organisms (Table 3) are capable of decolorizinga wide range of azo dyes (Fu and Viraraghavan, 2001). Manygenera of fungi have been employed either in living or inactivated form. Research on the fungal decolorization of dye wastewater has been performed in recent years. Several fungi with the capability to decolorize a wide range of dyes have been reported. For example, the white-rot fungi and brown-rot fungi are well-studied fungi groups with decolorization abilities (Singh *et al.*, 2014). White-rot fungi, such as *Phanerochaete chrysosporium, Trametes versicolor, Coriolus versicolor* and *Funalia trogii* have been reported to effectively decolorize various textile dyes. Decolorization abilities of some fungi, other than White-rot fungi, such as *Aspergillus niger, Rhizopus arrhizus* and *Rhizopus oryzae* were also reported for decolorization or absorb diverse dyes and possess excellent color removal capabilities (Taskin and Erdal2010; Zhou and Banks1991). The mechanism of fungal decolorization mainly involves two aspects biodegradation and biosorption (Vanhulle etal., 2008).The biodegradation capability of fungi is due to their extracellular, non-specific and non-selective enzyme system(Baccar *et al.*, 2011). Fungal enzyme production depends on nutrient limitations and their subsequent dye decolorization ability is achieved depending on the growth conditions (Kaushik and Malik 2009). Considering the complex environmental factors involved in the dye wastewater conditions, the screening of more fungi is necessary for use in dye decolorization.

Ligninolytic fungi have been studied as the possibleagents of biodegradation because their extracellular degradation systems are basically nonspecifific, a fact that allows the degradation of mixture of refractory substances (Kirk & Farrell 1987).The major enzymes associated with white-rotfungi are lignin peroxidase (EC 1.11.1.14)(LiP), manganese peroxidase (EC 1.11.1.13) (MnP) and laccase (EC1.10.3.2)(Lcc) (Vicuna 2000). Some of the white-rotfungi produce all these enzymes, while others produceonly one or two of them (Leonowicz *et al.*, 2001). Inmost cases, laccase-mediated dyedecolorization has been shown by many others (Rodriguez *et al.*, 1999; Pointing & Vrijmoed 2000; Kahraman and Yesilada 2001) and the activities of LiP (Young and Yu 1997) and MnP (Heinflfling *et al.*, 1998) also involved in decolorization of dyes. Phanerochaete chrysosporium decolorizes diffrent dyes such as Orange II, Tropaeolin O, Congo Red and Azure B in cultures medium and decolorization was determined by monitoring the decrease in absorbance at or near the wavelength maximum for each dye (Crips *et al.*, 1990). Heinflfling *et al.* (1997) reported that out of 18 fungal strains tested,only Bjerkandera adusta, Trametes versicolor and Phanerochaete chrysosporium were able to decolorizereactive orange 96, reactive blue 5, reactive violet 5, reactive blue 15 and reactive blue 38 dyes on agar plates. Wilkolazka *et al.* (2002) reported that among 115 testedfungi, 68 strains showed decolorization of the basic blue22 within 5–14 days on agar plate. A fungus *Cladosporium cladosporioides* isolated from coal sample as a laccase producing microorganism and decolorizes five different azo and triphenylmethane dyes like acid blue 193, acid black 210, crystal violet, reactive black B(S) and reactive black BL/LPR both on solid and in liquid broth medium. Culture broth of Cladosporium cladosporioides decolorized completely 100 mg/l of acid blue 193 in 8 days and the extracellular enzyme of decolorizes 564 mg of acid blue 193 on repeated addition within168 h without significant decline in the activity at optimum temperature 40°C, pH 5.6 and 4%sugar (Vijayakumar *et al.*, 2006). Laccase catalyzes the oxidation of a broad range of organic andinorganic substrates, including diphenols, polyphenols, diamines, aromatic amines, and ascorbate, via a one-electron transfer mechanism (Thurston 1994; Ullah *et al.*, 2000). Due to its low substrate specifificity, laccase can be usedin drug analysis, wine clarifification, bioremediation (Mayer and Staples 2002), paper-pulpbleaching, decolorization of synthetic dyes (Baldrian 2006) and biosensors (Vianello *et al.*, 2006). Recently, laccase was also reported to inhibit the activity of HIV-1 reverse transcriptase (Wang and Ng 2006). The practical applications of laccasein biotechnology have led to the need to expand the spectrum of microorganisms with laccase activities and the isolation of a novellaccase with different physicochemical and catalytic properties (Kiiskinen *et al.*, 2004). The decolorization of the mixture of two dyes from different classes (triphenylmethane brilliant green and azo Evans blue) by Pleurotus ostreatus (BWPH and MB), Gloeophyllum odoratum (DCa), RWP17 (Polyporus picipes) and Fusarium oxysporum (G1) were tested and significantly removed by all the strains that were tested with 96 h of experimental time (Przystas *et al.*, 2015). The white rot fungus Coriolopsis sp. was tested to decolorize four pigments of different colors or common backbones (Chen *et al.*, 2015) and Phanerochaete chrysosporium showed the decolorization ability for Acid Blue 62, Direct Red 80 and indigo dye (Faraco *et al.*, 2009; Sing *et al.*, 2010).

The Trametes versicolor decolorized more than 90% of 200 mg/L acid dyes (red 114, blue 62 and black 172) and reactive dyes (red 120, blue 4, orange 16 and black 5) within 6 days in the PDB medium. CBR43 decolorized 67% of 200 mg/L acid orange 7 within 9 days. The decolorization efficiencies for disperse dyes (red 1, orange 3 and black 1) were 51-80% within 9 days. The CBR43 could effectively decolorize high concentrations of acid blue 62 and acid black 172 (500-700 mg/L) at optimum temperature 28°C, pH 5, and 150 rpm in the PDB medium. This fungus has decolorizing activities of azo-type dyes as well as anthraquinone-type dyes and is one of promising bioresources for the decolorization of textile wastewater including various dyes (Yang *et al.* 2017). Legerska *et al.* (2018) reported the decolourization and detoxification of azo dyes (Orange 2, Acid Orange 6) by fungal laccase from Trametes versicolor. The laccase treatment was more effective for the Orange 2 decolourization, the toxicity of both monoazo dye solutions became less toxic for the prokaryote growth.

The phytotoxicity of Orange 2 and Acid Orange 6 solutions after laccase treatment was decreased in the range of 41.2-64.3%. Also, the photoxicity, as measured by the production of chlorophylls a and b by Chlorella vulgaris and Microcystis aeruginosa, was decreased by laccase treatment of selected monoazo dyes. Our results show that different dyes can be decolorized and detoxified by laccase from T. versicolor in a single step (Legerska *et al.*, 2018). Hao *et al.*, (2018) has isolated three laccase-producing fungus strains from Taxus rhizosphere and Myrotheium verrucaria strain DJTU-sh7 had the highest laccase activity of 216.2 U/ml, which was increased to above 300 U/ml after optimization. The DJTU-sh7-containing fungal consortium displayed the robust decolorizing ability and both color removal efficiency, chemical oxygen demand were increased in the consortium mediated biotransformation. Based on the successful laboratory results, efforts should now be made to scale-up and apply fungal decolourization techniques in real industrial effluents. While on one hand recent advances like enzyme immobilization may help in enhancing the efficiency, search for robust, alkaline and heat tolerant strains might make the process more economical and viable.

Table 1: Different physical and chemical methods for dye removal from textile effluent with its advantages and disadvantages (Robinson *et al.*, 2002).

Physical/chemical method	Advantages	Disadvantages
Fentons reagent	Effective decolaration of soluble and insoluble dyes	Sludge generation
Ozonation	Applied in gaseous state, no alteration of volume	Short half life (20 min)
Photochemical	No sludge production	Formation of by-products
Sodium hypochlorite	Initiates and accelerate azo bond Cleavage	Release of aromatic amines
Electrochemical destruction	Break-down compounds are nonhazardous	High electricity consumption
Activated carbon	Good removal of wide variety of dyes	Very expensive
Peat	Good adsorbent due to cellular structure	Specific surface area for adsorption are lower than activated carbon
Wood chips	Good sorption capacity for acidic dyes	Require long retention time
Silica gel	Effective for basic dye removal	Side reactions prevent commercial application
Membrane filtration	Removal all types of dyes	Concentrated sludge production
Ion-exchange	No adsorbent loss due to regeneration	Not effective for all dyes
Irradiation	Effective oxidation at laboratory scale	Requires high concentrations of dissolved oxygen
Electrokinetic coagulation	Economically feasible	High sludge production

Table 2: Bacterial decolorization of dyes.

Dyes	Decolorization (%)	Reference
Mixture of dyes	87	Saratale *et al.*, (2013)
Amaranth, Acid Orange 52, Direct Blue 71	efficient	Liu *et al.*, (2013)
Brown 3REL (B3REL), SRR, Remazol Red (RR), Direct Red 2B (DR2B)and Malachite Green (MG)	100	Kabra *et al.*, (2013)
Sulphonated Azo dyes, Acid Orange 7 (AO7) and Acid Red 88 (AR88)	~100	De los Cobos Vasconcelos *et al.*, (2012)
Mixture of dyes	high	Naik *et al.*, (2012)

Dyes	Decolorization (%)	Reference
Orange P3R, Yellow P3R, Blue H5R, Violet P3R, Brown P5R, Black V3R, Orange P2R	47.24	Jayan *et al.*, (2011)
Remazol Red, Rubine GFL, Brown 3REL, Scarlet RR, Golden Yellow HER, Methyl Red, Brilliant Blue GL	87	Kurade *et al.*, (2011)
8 textile dyes	89	Joshi *et al.*, (2010)
Congo red, Bordeaux, Ranocid Fast Blue and Blue BCC	50-60	Tony *et al.*, (2009)
16 Azo dyes	90	Joshi *et al.*, (2008)
Acid Red 88, Reactive Black 5, Direct Red 81, and Disperse Orange 3	100	Khalid *et al.*, (2008
Azo dyes	-	Asad *et al.*, (2007)
Naphthalene-containing sulfonated azo dyes Amaranth , Fast Red E and Ponceau S	100	Vijaykumar *et al.*, (2007)
Red RB, Remazol Red, Remazol Blue, Remazol Violet, Remazol Yellow, Golden Yellow, Remazol Orange, Remazol Black	95	Padmavathy *et al.*, (2003)

Table 3: Fungal decolorization of dyes.

Dyes	Decolorization (%)	Reference
Azo–Anthraquinone dye mixture (Azure B, Congo Red, Trypan Blue and Remazol Brilliant Blue R)	74.93	Taha *et al.*, (2014)
Triarylmethane dye (Brilliant green) and Diazo dye (Evans blue)	80	Przystas *et al.*, (2013)
Yellow FG, Red 3BS, Orange 3R, Blue RSP, Black B and remazol turquoise blue	82	Idris *et al.*, (2013)
Reactive azo dyes (red, black and orange II)	88	Ambrósio *et al.*, (2012)
Remazol Red, Golden Yellow HER, Rubine GFR, Scarlet RR, Methyl Red, Brown 3REL, Brilliant Blue	88	Waghmode *et al.*, (2011)
Direct Red-80 and Mordant Blue-9	77–97	Pakshirajan and Singh (2010)
Reactive blue 21, Reactive black 5 and Reactive orange 13	60-66	Nordstrom *et al.*, (2008)
Acid blue 193, Acid Black 210	100	Viajayakumar *et al.*, 2006

Dyes	Decolorization (%)	Reference
Remazol Brilliant Orange 1, Levafix Gold Yellow 10, Procion Yellow 14, Drimaren Brilliant Blue 17, Remazol Brilliant Blue 18, Cibacron Black 55, Procion Black 59, Drimaren Turquoise Blue 62, Drimaren Brilliant Red 67, and Remazol Red 75	80-90	Machado *et al.*, (2006)
Mixtures of 4 reactive textile dyes, azo and anthraquinone dyes	90	Harazono and Nakamura, (2005)
Orange , Reactive Black , Reactive Red	88	Ambrosio and Camx-pos-Takaki, (2004)
ProcionOrange MX-2R (C.I. Reactive Orange 4), Remazol Red 3B (C.I. Reactive Red 23) and Remazol Black GF (C.I. Reactive Black 5)	97	Amaral *et al.*, (2004)
Meta or para aminobenzoic or amino-sul-Phonic acids as diazo components and two fungal bioaccessible groups present in lignin structure, guaiacol or syringol, as coupling components	100	Martins *et al.*, (2003)

References

Amaral, P F F., Fernandes, D L A., Tavares, A P M.,and Xavier,A B M R. (2004). Decolorization of dyes from texti lewastewater by Trametes versicolor. Environ. Technol.25:1313-1320.

Ambrosio, ST., and Takaki, GMC. (2004). Decolorization ofreactive azo dyes by Cunninghamellaelegans UCP 542 underco-metabolic conditions. *Bioresour.* Technol.91:69-75.

Ambrosio, ST., Vilar Junior, J C., da Silva, C A A.,and Okada, K.(2012). A biosorption isotherm model for the removal ofreactive azo dyes by inactivated mycelia of *Cunninghamellaelegans* UCP542. Molecules.17:452-462.

Asad, S., Amoozegar, MA., Pourbabaee, A., Sarbolouki, MN., and Dastgheib, S M M. (2007).Decolorization of textile azodyes by newly isolated halophilic and halotolerant bacteria. *Bioresour. Technol.* 98:2082-2088.

Azmi, W., Sani, R K., and Banerjee, UC. (1998). *Biodegradationof triphenylmethane* dyes. Enzyme Microb. Tech. 22(3):185-191.

Baccar, R., Blanquez, P., Bouzid, J., Feki, M., Attiya, H., and Sarra, M. (2011). Decolorization of a tannery dye: from fungal screening to bioreactor application. *Biochem Eng J.* 56(3):184–189.

Baldrian, P. (2006). Fungal laccases—occurrence and properties. FEMS Microbiol Rev. 30:215–242.

Beydilli, M. I., Pavolsathis, S G., and Tincher, W C. (1998).Decolorization and toxicity screening of selected reactiveazo dyes under methanogenic condition. *Water Sci. Tech.* 38(4-5): 225-232.

Chen, H.,Xu, H., Heinze, T M., and Cerniglia, C E. (2009). Decolorization of water and oil-soluble azo dyes by Lactobacillus acidophilus and Lactobacillus fermentum. *J. Ind. Microbiol. Biotechnol.* 36(12):1459–1466.

Chen, SH., Yien,T., and Ting, AS. (2015). Biodecolorization and biodegradation potential of recalcitrant triphenylmethane dyes by Coriolopsis sp. isolated from compost. *J. Environ. Manage.*150:274–280.

Cheriaa, J., Khaireddine, M., Rouabhia, M., and Bakhrouf, A. (2012). Removal of Triphenylmethane Dyes by Bacterial Consortium. *Scientific World Journal.* 2012: 512454.

Crips, C., Bumpus, J., and Aust, S. (1990). Biodegradation of Azo and Heterocyclic Dyes by Phanerochaete chrysosporium. *Appl. Environ. Microbiol.*56(4):1114-1118.

De los Cobos-Vasconcelos, D., Ruiz-Ordaz, N., Galíndez-Mayer, J., Poggi-Varaldo, H., Juàrez-Ramírez, C., and Aarón, L.-M. (2011). Aerobic biodegradation of a mixture of sulfonated azo dyes by a bacterial consortium immobilized in a two-stage sparged packed-bed biofilm reactor. *Eng. Life Sci.*12(1):39–48.

Faraco, V., Pezzella, C., and Giardina, P. (2009). Decolourization of textile dyes by the white-rot fungi Phanerochaete chrysosporium and Pleurotus ostreatus. *J. Chem. Technol. Biotechnol.*84:414–419.

Fu, Y., and Viraraghavan, T. (2001). Fungal decolorization of dye wastewater: a review. *Bioresour Technol.* 79:251–262.

Govindwar, SP., Kurade, MB., Tamboli, DP., Kabra, AN., and Kim, PJ. (2014). Waghmode TR. Decolorization and degradation of xenobiotic azo dye Reactive Yellow-84A and textile effluent by *Galactomyces geotrichum. Chemosphere.* 109:234-8.

Gueu, S., Yao, B., Adouby, K.,and Ado, G. (2007). Kinetics andthermodynamics study of lead adsorption on to activatedcarbons from coconut and seed hull of the palm tree. *Int.J. Environ. Sci. Tech.* 4(1):11-17.

Hao, D C., Song, S M., Cheng, Y., Qin, Z Q., Ge, G B., An, B L., and Xia, P G. (2018). Functional and Transcriptomic Characterization of a Dye-decolorizing Fungus from Taxus Rhizosphere. *Polish J. Microb.* 67(4):417–429.

Harazono, K., and Nakamura, K. (2005). Decolorization ofmixtures of different reactive textile dyes by the whiterotbasidiomycete Phanerochaete sordida and inhibitory effectof polyvinyl alcohol. *Chemosphere.* 59:63-68.

Heinflfling, A., Martinez, MJ., Martinez, AT., Bergbauer, M.,and Szewzyl, U. (1998). Transformation of industrial dyes by manganeseperoxidase from Bjerkandera adusta and Pleurotus eryngii in amanganese-dependent reaction. *Appl. and Environ. Microb.*64:2788–2793.

Heinfling, A., Bergbauer, M., and Szewzyk, U.(1997). Biodegradation of azo and phthalocyanine dyes by Trametes versicolor and Bjerkandera adusta. *Appl. Microbiol. Biotechnol.* 48:261–266.

Idris, A., Suhaimi, MS., Zain, NAM., Rashid, R.,and Othman,N. (2014). Discoloration of aqueous textile dyes solutionby Phanerochaete chrysosporium immobilized in modifiedPVA matrix. Desalination and Water Treatment.52(34-36):6694-6702.

Jayan, MA., Maragatham, NR.,and Saravanan, J. (2011). *Decolorization* and physico chemical analysis of textile azodye by Bacillus. *Int. J. Appl. Bioeng.*5:35-39.

Joshi, SM., Inamdar, SA., Telke, AA., Tamboli, DP., and Govindwar, SP. (2010). Exploring the potential of naturalbacterial consortium to degrade mixture of dyes and textileeffluent. *Int. Biodeterioration and Biodegradation.* 64:622-628.

Joshi, T., Iyengar, L., Singh, K., and Garg, S. (2008). Isolation, identification and application of novel bacterial consortiumTJ-1 for the decolourization of structurally different azodyes. *Bioresour. Technol.* 99:7115-7121.

Kabra, AN., Khandare, RV.,and Govindwar, SP. (2013).Development of a bioreactor for remediation of textileeffluent and dye mixture: *A plant–bacterial synergisticstrategy.* Water Res.47:1035-1048.

Kahraman, S.,and Yesilada, O. (2001). Industrial and agricultural wastesas substrates for Laccase production by white-rot fungi. Folia Microb.46:133–136.

Kaushik, P., Malik, A. (2009). Fungal dye decolourization: recent advances and future potential. Environ Int. 35(1):127–141.

Khalid, A., Arshad, M.,and Crowley, DE. (2008). Accelerateddecolorization of structurally different azo dyes by newlyisolated bacterial strains. *Appl. Microbiol. Biotech.*78:361-369.

Khandare, R V., Kabra, A N., Awate, A V., and Govindwar, S P. (2013). Synergistic degradation of diazo dye Direct Red 5B by Portulaca grandiflora and Pseudomonas putida. *Int. J. Environ. Sci. Technol.*10:1039–1050.

Kiiskinen, LL., Rättö, M., and Kruus, K. (2004). Screening for novel laccaseproducing microbes.J. Appl. Microbiol.97:640–646.

Kirk, TK.,and Farrell, R. (1987). Enzymatic "combustion" the microbialdegradation of lignin. Annual Review of Microb.41:465–505 .

Kolekar, YM., Konde, PD., Markad, VL., Kulkarni, SV., and Chaudhari, AU. (2013). Effective bioremoval anddetoxification of textile dye mixture by Alishewanella sp.KMK6. Appl. Microbiol. Biotech.97:881-889.

Kumar, MA., Kumar, VV., Ponnusamy, R., Daniel, FP., Seenuvasan, M., Anuradha, D., and Sivanesane, S. (2015). Concomitant mineralization and detoxification of Acid Red 88 by an indigenousacclimated mixed culture. Environ. Progress Sustain Energy.34:1455–1466.

Kurade, MB., Waghmode, TR.,and Govindwar, SP. (2011).Preferential biodegradation of structurally dissimilar dyesfrom a mixture by Brevibacilluslaterosporus. J. Hazard.Mater.192:1746-1755.

Legerská, B., Chmelová, D., and Ondrejovič, M. (2018). Decolourization and detoxification of monoazo dyes by laccase from the white-rot fungusTrametes versicolor. *J. Biotechnol.* 285:84-90.

Leonowicz, A., Cho, NS., Luterek, J., Wilkolazka, A., WojtasWasilewska, M., Matuszewska, A., Hofrichter, M., Wesen-Berg,D.,and Rogalski, J. (2001). Fungal Laccase: properties and activity onlignin. *J. ofBasic Microb.*41:185–227.

Liu, G., Zhou, J., Meng, X., Fu, SQ., Wang, J., Jin, R.,and Lv, H.(2013). Decolorization of azo dyes by marine Shewanellastrains under saline conditions. *Appl. Microbiol. Biotech.*97:4187-4197.

Liu, W., You, Y., Sun, D., Wang, S., Zhu, J., and Liu, C. (2018). Decolorization and detoxification of water-insoluble Sudan dye by Shewanella putrefaciens CN32 co-cultured with Bacillus circulans BWL1061.Ecotoxicol Environ Saf. 30(166):11-17.

Machado, KM., Compart, LC., Morais, RO., Rosa, LH., and Santos,MH. (2006). Biodegradation of reactive textile dyes bybasidiomycetous fungi from Brazilian ecosystems. *Brazilian J. Microbiol.*37: 481-487.

Manjinder, SK., Harvinder, SS., Deepak K S., Bhupnder SC., and Swapndeep SC. (2005). Decolourization of various azo dyes by bacterial consortium. Dyes and Pigments.67:55-61.

Martins, MAM., Lima, N., Silvestre, AJ., and Queiroz, MJ.(2003). Comparative studies of fungal degradation of singleor mixed bioaccessible reactive azo dyes. *Chemosphere*. 52:967-973.

Mayer, AM., and Staples, RC. (2002). Laccase: new functions for an old enzyme. Phytochemistry. 60:551–65.

McMullan, G., Meehan, C., Connely, A., Kirby, N., Robinson, T., Marchant, R., and Smyth, WF. (2001). Microbial decolourization and degradation of textile dyes. Appl. Microb. Biotechnol.56:81-88.

Naik, C., and Singh, C.R. (2012). Isolation screening anddevelopment of Bacillus sp. with decolorization anddegradation capabilities towards reactive dyes and textileeffluents. *Recent Res. Sci.* Tech.4:No-5.

Nordstrom, F., Terrazas, E., and Welander, U. (2008).Decolorization of a mixture of textile dyes using Bjerkanderasp. Bol 13. Environ. Tech.29:921-929.

Padamavathy, S. (2003). Aerobic decolorization of reactiveazo dyes in presence of various co substrates. Chemicaland Biochem. Eng. Quarterly. 17:147-152.

Pakshi rajan, K., and Singh, S. (2010). Decolorizat ion ofsynthetic wastewater containing azo dyes in a batchoperatedrotating biological contactor reactor with the immobilizedfungus Phanerochaete chrysosporium. Ind. Eng. Chem. Res.49:7484-7487.

Pandey, A., Singh, P., and Iyengar, L. (2007). Bacterial decolorization and degradation of azo dyes. Int. Biodeter. Biodegrad.59:73–84.

Pointing, SB., and Vrijmoed, LLP. (2000). Decolorization of azo and triphenylmethane dyes by Picnoporus sanguineus producing Laccase as the sole phenol oxidase. World J. of Microb andBiotech.16:317–318.

Przystas, W., Godlewska, E Z.,and Grabinska, E S. (2013).Effectiveness of dyes removal by mixed fungal cultures andtoxicity of their metabolites. Water Air Soil Pollut.224:1-9.

Przystas, W., Zablocka-Godlewska, E., and Grabinska-Sota, E. (2015). Efficacy of fungal decolorization of a mixture of dyes belonging to different classes. Brazilian J. Microb. 46(2):415-424.

Robinson, T., Chandran, B., and Nigam, P. (2002). Removal of dyes from an artificial textile dye effluent by two agricultural residue, corncob and barley husk. Environment Int. 28(1-2):29-33.

Rodríguez, C S., and Toca, H JL. (2006). Industrial and biotechnological applications of laccases: a review. Biotechnol Adv. 24(5):500–513.

Rodriguez, E., Pickard, MA.,and Vazquez-Duhalt, R. (1999). Industrialdye decolorization by laccases from ligninolytic fungi. Curr. Microb. 38:27–32.

Saratale, RG., Gandhi, SS., Purankar, MV., Kurade, MB., (2013). Decolorization and detoxification of sulfonated azodye CI Remazol Red and textile effluent by isolatedLysinibacillus sp. RGS. J. Biosci. Bioeng.115:658-667.

Singh, A P., and Singh, T. (2014). *Biotechnological* applications of wood-rotting fungi: a review. *Biomass Bioenergy*. 62:198–206.

Singh, S., Pakshirajan, K., and Daverey, A. (2010). Enhanced decolourization of Direct Red-80 dye by the white rot fungus Phanerochaete chrysosporium employing sequential design of experiments. Biodegradation.21:501–511.

Singh, L., and Singh, VP. (2012). Microbial decolourization of textile dyes by the fungus Trichoderma harzianum. *J Pure and Appl Microbiol*. 6(4):1829–1833.

Spadaro, J T., Gold, M H., and Renganathan, V. (1992). Degradation of azo dyes by the lignin degrading fungus Phanerochaete chrysosporium. Appl. Environ. Microb. 58(8):2397-2401.

Taha, M., Adetutu, E M., Shahsavari, E., Smith, A T.,and Ball, AS. (2014). Azo and anthraquinone dye mixture decolourizationat elevated temperature and concentration by a newly isolatedthermophilic fungus, Thermomucorindicae-seudaticae. *J.Environ. Chem.* Eng.2:415–423.

Tamboli, D P., Kurade, M B., Waghmode, T R., Joshi, S M., and Govindwar, S P. (2010). Exploring the ability of Sphingobacterium sp. ATM to degrade textile dye direct blue GLL,mixture of dyes and textile effluent and production ofpolyhydroxyhexadecanoic acid using waste biomassgenerated after dye degradation. J. Hazard. Mater. 182:169-176.

Taskin, M., and Erdal, S. (2010). Reactive dye bioaccumulation by fungus Aspergillus niger isolated from the effluent of sugar fabric-contaminated soil. Toxic. Ind. Health.26:239-247.

Thurston, CF. (1994). The structure and function of fungal laccase. Microbiology. 140:19–26.

Tony, B D., Goya, D.,and Khanna, S. (2009). Decolorization of textile azo dyes by aerobic bacterialconsortium. Int. Biodeterioration &Biodegradation.63:462-469.

Ullah, MA., Bedford, CT., and Evans, CS. (2000). Reactions of pentachlorophenol with laccasefrom Coriolus versicolor. Appl. Micrbiol. Biotechnol.53:230–234.

Vanhulle, S., Trovaslet, M., Enaud, E. (2008). Decolorization, cytotoxicity, and genotoxicity reduction during a combined ozonation/fungal treatment of dye-contaminated wastewater. *Environ Sci Technol.* 42(2):584–589.

Vianello, F., Ragusa, S., Cambria, MT., and Rigo, A A.(2006). high sensitivity amperometric biosensor using laccase as biorecognition element. *Biosens Bioelectron.* 21:2155–2160.

Vicuna, R. (2000). Ligninolysis. A very peculiar microbial process. *Molecular Biotech.*14:173–176.

Vijaykumar, M H., Vaishampayan, P A., Shouche, Y S., and Karegoudar, T B. (2007). Decolour ization ofnaphthalene-containing sulfonated azo dyes by Kerstersiasp.Strain VKY1. *Enzyme and Microbial. Technol.*40:204-211.

Vijaykumar, M H., Veeranagouda, Y., Neelakanteshwar,K., and Karegoudar, T B. (2006). Decolorization of 1:2 metal complex dye Acid blue 193 by a newly isolated fungus,Cladosporium cladosporioides. World J. of Microb. Biotech.22:157–162.

Waghmode, T R., Kurade, M B.,and Govindwar, S P. (2011). Timedependent degradation of mixture of structurally different azoand non azo dyes by using Galactomycesgeotrichum MTCC1360. *Int. Biodeterioration and Biodegradation.* 65:479-486.

Wang, HX., and Ng, TB. (2006). Purifification of a laccase from fruiting bodies of the mushroom Pleurotus eryngii. Appl. Microbiol. Biotechnol.69:521–525.

Wilkolazka, AJ., Rdest, JK., Malarczyk, E., Wardas, W., and Leonowicz, A. (2002). Fungi and their ability to decolorize azoand anthraquinonic dyes. Enzyme and Microb. Technol. 30:566–572.

Xu, X. R., Li, H B., Wang, W H., and Gu, J D. (2005).Decolorization of dyes and textile was tewater by potassiumpermanganate. Chemosphere.(59):893-898.

Yang, SO, Sodaneath, H., Lee, JI., Jung, H., Choi, JH., Ryu, HW., and Cho, KS. (2017). Decolorization of acid, disperse and reactive dyes by Trametes versicolor CBR43.J. Environ. Sci. Health. A Tox. Hazard. Subst. Environ. Eng. 52(9):862-872.

Young, L., and J. Yu. (1997). Ligninase catalyzed decolorization of synthetic dyes. Water Res. 31:1187–1193.

Zhou, JL., and Banks, CJ. (1991). Removal of humic acid fractions by Rhizopus arrhizus: Uptake and kinetic studies. Environ. Technol.12:859-869.

Innovations in Biochemical Techniques (2020) : Page no. 153-173
ASTRAL INTERNATIONAL (P) LTD., New Delhi - 110002

Chapter 12

Causes of Cancer and their Different Types of Therapy

Proma Chakraborty

School of Sciences, Department of Life Sciences, Garden City University Bengaluru, Karnataka, India

Email: proma.c@gardencitycollege.edu

The word "Cancer" is derived from a Greek word called "Cancrum" which means crab. The movement of the crab has been compared with the uncontrolled proliferation of metastatic tumour cells. There are several factors which are responsible for neoplastic conversion some of them are listed below.

Causes of Cancer

1. **Gene Mutation:** *Four classes of normal regulatory genes—the growth-promoting protooncogenes, the growth-inhibiting tumor suppressor genes, genes that regulate programmed cell death (apoptosis), and genes involved in DNA repair—are the principal targets of genetic damage that are responsible for cancer.* (Santarosa; 2004)

   (*i*) **Growth Promoting proto-oncogenes:** Cell possess proto-oncogenes, which encode protein that carry out normal activities of the cell and promote normal cell growth. They are known as positive regulators of cell cycle. Proto oncogene mutation by point substitution, proviral insertion, amplification or dysregulation converts them into tumour causing oncogenes. Oncogenes encode proteins that promote loss of growth control and transform the cell to a malignant or neoplastic state. Thus oncogenes are genes whose action promotes cell proliferation.

   The proteins encoded by oncogenes are called oncoproteins or transforming proteins. These proteins are highly conserved in evolution. The proteins encoded by oncogenes have been classified into six broad categories on the basis of enzymatic activity and the localization of proteins.

   Class I: Extracellular growth factors and hormones – These include the products of sis and int – 2 oncogenes.

   Class II: Transmembrane cell growth factor surface receptors – Tyrosine –specific protein kinases. These proteins of an extracellular Ligand binding domain and intacellular enzymatic domain which propagates signals by phosphorylating specific substrate proteins on tyrosine residue, Example: erb A and fms gene products.

Class III: Membrane associated G-proteins - intracellular signal transducers these proteins bind GTP and play important roles in cellular signal transduction. Example: Ras protein

Class IV: **Intracellular tyrosin specific protein kinases** – these proteins amplify incoming signals. Examples – src and abl proteins.

Class V: **Cytosolic serine/threonine – specific protein kinase** – these proteins act as intermediary components of signal transduction chains. Some are activated through a cytoplasmic process and phosphorylate nuclear target proteins (bridge between cytoplasm and nucleus). Examples of cytoplasmic proteins are the mos and raf proteins.

Class VI: **Nuclear oncoproteins including transcriptional regulators** – these are the only oncogene products localized to the cell nucleus. They bind to specific DNA sequences and control the rate of transcription of cellular genes. Example are the myc, fos, jun and erbA gene products. (C.B.Powar)

Mechanisms converting proto-oncogenes to cancer causing oncogenes

- Point Mutation
- Proviral Insertion : The activation of the c-myc gene by proviral insertion includes three mechanisms
  - ❑ Insertion in Intron – 1between exons E1 and E2 has a promoter effect. The right hand LTR which normally functions as a terminator now acts as an efficient promoter
  - ❑ Insertion in Intron 1, but in the reverse direction has an enhancer effect. In this orientation, the LTR does not function as a promoter but provides an enhancer that acts on an upstream sequence that resembles a promoter
  - ❑ Insertion 3′ (downstream) of exon 3 has an enhancer effect through LTR
- Deletion
- Translocation
- Amplification (Powar)

(ii) **Tumour suppressor genes or anti-oncogenes:** Normal cells contain genes on their chromosomes that suppress unregulated cell growth or proliferation. These genes are called tumour suppressor genes (TSGs). TSGs encode proteins that restrain cell growth and prevent cells from becoming mutants. The normal products of TSGs have an inhibitory effect on cell growth and division. They are commonly known as negative regulators of cell cycle. In certain cancer, specific regions are deleted from both homologues resulting in deletion of both alleles of TSG. Inactivation of the TSG alleles results in the loss of the inhibiting activity. This in turn results in unregulated cell proliferation leading to cancer.

Somatic mutation of one allele of a TSG results in heterozygosity at that locus. This usually does not have significant consequences, and there is normal cell growth control. The normal allele codes for sufficient gene products for normal function. In some individuals the cells have inherited loss of function of one allele of the TSG with the other allele remaining functionally normal. Such individuals do not develop tumours. They are the potential carriers. Only when a mutation takes place in the remaining normal allele there will be uncontrolled cell growth. The mutation or loss of both alleles of TSG is necessary for a cell to lose growth control. Such cell will lack any copy of the wild type allele and protein encoded will therefore be inactive. Thus tumour-suppressor mutations that are found in tumour cells are recessive.

Mutated TSG shows gain of functional mutation. Instead of suppressing cell division the mutant version will promote the proliferation of cells.

In case of oncogenes, however, mutation of only one allele of a proto-oncogene, converting it into oncogenes, is enough for the cell to lose growth control. The oncogenes mutation is therefore dominant. (Ana Maria Abreu Velez; 2015).

(iii) **Genes that regulate programmed cell death (apoptosis):** Failure in apoptosis, or programmed cell death, is one of the significant processes in cancer development and progression. Apoptosis occurs through two pathways: the intrinsic, mitochondrial pathway, which is initiated by intracellular stresses and the extrinsic, death-receptor pathway, which is initiated by binding of cell surface receptors with specific ligands. The intrinsic pathway is negatively regulated by anti-apoptotic proteins, called the BCL-2 family. High expression of BCL – 2 prevents cell death. The extrinsic apoptotic pathway is induced through a specific ligand, such as Apo2L/TRAIL, binding to its cell surface receptor. In most cell types, the extrinsic pathway converges with the intrinsic pathway to induce apoptosis, which involves leakage of cytochrome c from mitochondrial membrane through pore formation. Cytochrome C forms a complex with APAF (Apoptotic protease activating factor) and induces activation of proteolytic enzymes, called caspases, leading to the destruction of the cells.

Tumor cells can acquire resistance to apoptosis by the expression of anti-apoptotic proteins such as Bcl-2 or by the down-regulation the expression of pro-apoptotic proteins such as Bax. Expression of Bcl-2 and Bax are inversely proportional to one another. In a normal cell which is not undergoing apoptosis will have high expression of Bcl-2 and low expression of Bax. In a dying cell the scenario is just the opposite Bcl- 2 will be down regulated and Bax will be upregulated. The expression of both Bcl-2 and Bax is regulated by the *p53* tumor suppressor gene. Certain forms of human B cell lymphoma have overexpression of Bcl-2, which prevents the cell from undergoing apoptosis. (Zhang; 2007) (*iv*) **Mutator genes and DNA repair:** These genes are required for the fidelity of replication and for maintaining the integrity of the genome. When there is mutation in mutator genes it results in loss of their normal functions and the cells get prone to accumulation of mutational errors. During DNA replication new stands are synthesized by coping complementary bases from the template. The replication system has high fidelity with very few errors. There are cases where errors in replication do occur due to environmental factors that lead to damaged DNA. Under such circumstances DNA repair mechanisms are switched on to repair such damages. However the repair system can become faulty through inherited or acquired mutations. With repeated cell divisions these mutations can accumulate throughout the genome. If these mutations involve TSGs or oncogenes, the chances of malignant transformation increase. (Lawrence, 2003)

2. **Viruses and Human Cancer:** Members of six distinct families of animal viruses, called tumor viruses, are capable of causing cancer. Viruses belonging to five of these families have DNA as their genetic material and are referred to as DNA tumor viruses. Members of the sixth family of tumor viruses commonly known as retroviruses, have RNA as genetic material and they replicate via synthesis of a DNA provirus in infected cells.

   The viruses that cause human cancer include hepatitis B virus (liver cancer), papillomaviruses (cervical and other anogenital cancers), Epstein-Barr virus (Burkitt's lymphoma and nasopharyngeal carcinoma), Kaposi's sarcoma-associated herpesvirus (Kaposi's sarcoma), and human T-cell lymphotropic virus (adult T-cell leukemia). In addition, HIV is indirectly responsible for the cancers that develop in AIDS patients as a result of immunodeficiency, and hepatitis C virus (an RNA virus) is an indirect cause of liver cancers resulting from chronic tissue damage. (Powar)

3. **Exposure to carcinogens (cancer inducing agents)**

   (*i*) **Radiation carcinogen:** Ionizing and non ionizing radiation

   (a) **Ionizing radiations** are so called because they cause ionization in the atoms present in their path of penetration through living tissues. The high energy radiations collide with atoms and cause the release of electrons leaving positively charged free radicals or ions. The electrons kicked away by ionizing radiation also behave in the same manner and in turn cause release of electrons from other atoms. The net result is formation of "core of ions" along their path of entry through living tissue. These ions undergo many chemical reactions to achieve their stable configuration. During these chemical reactions they cause mutations.

Ionization Effects

When the initial ionization event begins with water, to form free radicals (a highly reactive chemical species with an unpaired electron in its valance shell), that cause a cascade of biological responses in macromolecules, the mechanism is collectively called an indirect effect. The primary mechanism of biological damage to macromolecules from ionizing radiation is an indirect interaction that begins with the ***radiolysis*** of water.

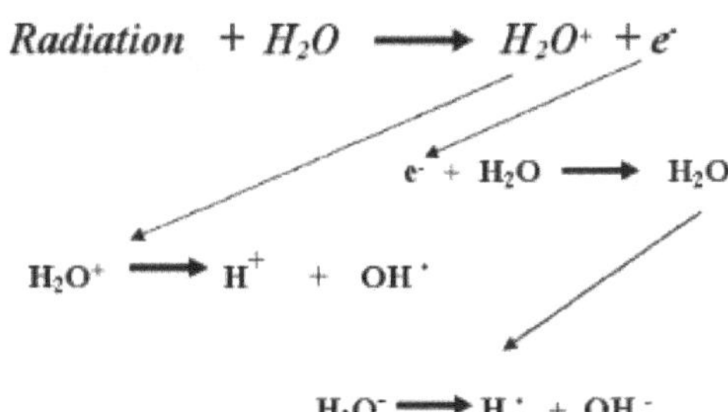

Ionization of water molecules cause them to split by a process called radiolysis. The event triggers a cascade of chemical reactions that result in the formation of free radicals. Free radicals are highly reactive particles which can cause subsequent DNA damage.

The net products of radiolysis of water molecules are the formation of highly reactive free radicals, namely a ***hydrogen free radical*** **(H˙)**, and a ***hydroxyl free radical*** **(OH˙)**. The third type of free radical from radiolysis of water is formed when the hydrogen free radical interacts with oxygen to form a highly reactive species called ***hydroperoxyl radical*** **($HO_2^{\cdot}$)**; these three free radicals are the results of ionization of water molecules and radiolysis. The free electron (e-) combines with water and forms the negative water molecule called "heavy water," which is a precursor to the hydroxyl radical **(OH˙)**. (H. Dertinger; 1969)

Chemical species formed by radiolysis which is given below:

1. **Two hydroxyl radical can combine to form hydrogen peroxide (H_2O_2) that is converted back to water by the organelle called the peroxisome:**

$$OH^{\cdot} + OH^{\cdot} \longrightarrow H_2O_2$$

2. **The hydrogen radical and the hydroxyl radical can combine to form water:**

$$H^{\cdot} + OH^{\cdot} \longrightarrow H_2O$$

3. **The hydrogen ion and hydroxyl ion can combine to form water:**

$$H^{+} + OH^{-} \longrightarrow H_2O$$

4. **The hydrogen free radical can combine with molecular oxygen to form a highly reactive hydroperoxyl radical which continues the chain of radical damage to biomolecules:**

$$H^{\cdot} + O_2 \longrightarrow HO_2^{\cdot}$$

Ionizing radiation cause breaks in sugar phosphate backbone of DNA and thus causing chromosomal mutations such as deletions.

(b) **Non-ionizing radiation** is the term given to radiation in the part of the electromagnetic spectrum where there is insufficient energy to cause ionization. It only raises the energy level of an electron so that it moves into an outer orbit representing a higher energy level of the same atom. Consequently such an atom has an unpaired electron in two of its orbit and is much more reactive than the normal atoms; production of such atoms is called excitation. The exited atom is called photoproduct which can cause mutation. (Matt Jackson ; 2014).

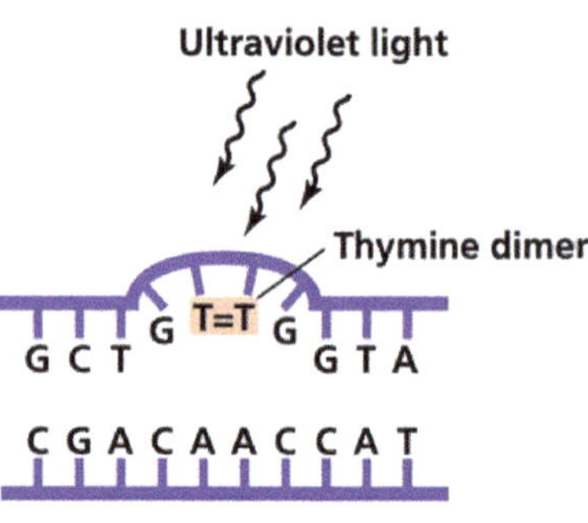

Formation of pyrimidine dimers: Non-ionizing radiation such as ultraviolet light causes the breaking of bonds between purines and pyrimindines. When two pyrimidine molecules of the same type (T or C) are adjacent to one another on a nucleoside they tend to form dimers. These **pyrimidine dimers** distort the sugar phosphate backbone by displacement of hydrogen bonds and thus prevent proper replication and transcription.

Pyrimidine dimer induced by UV light. In this figure thymine has been used as an example. Cytosine may form a similar dimer.

Formation of Pyrimidine Hydrates: Formation of cytosine photohydrate (6-hydroxy-5,6-dihydrocytosine) as a result of photohydration reaction. During hydration the double bond between 4 and 5 carbon of cytosine is disrupted followed by addition of –H and –OH group of water molecule to 4 and 5 carbon atoms respectively. (Rastogi RP, 2010)

NH_2 NH_2 H UV N N O N O N OH

Cytocine Cytocine hydrate

(*ii*) Chemical carcinogen

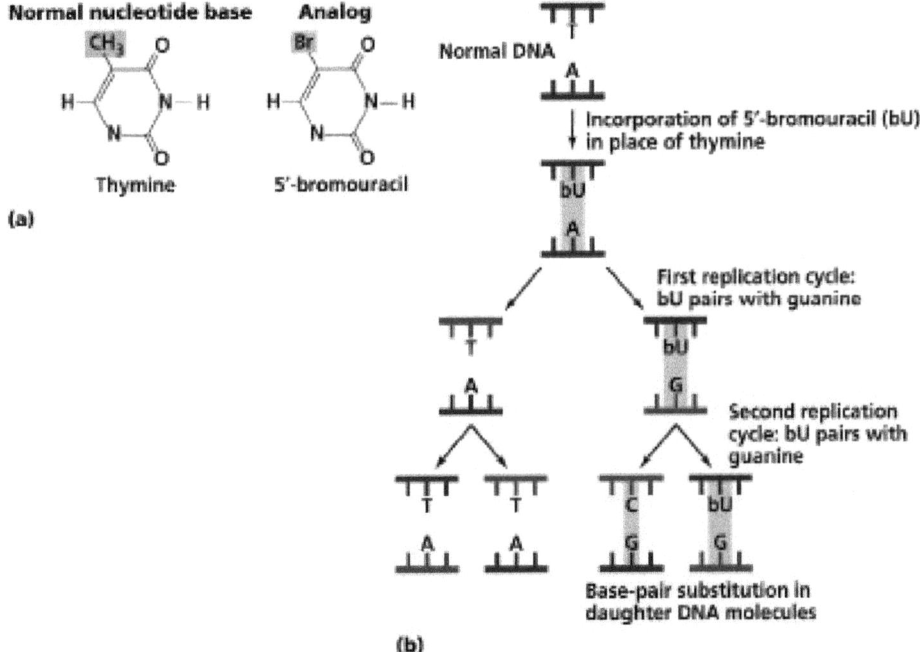

Base analogs have a chemical structure similar to a normal nucleotide (as for example 5′-bromouracil resembles thymine) and compete with the normal nucleotide during DNA replication thus causing point mutations. The presence of Br in the 5 position of 5′-bromouracil has the same effect on its base pairing behaviour as that of CH_3 in the same position of thymine. Therefore 5BU behaves like thymine and usually base pairs with adenine. The presence of bromine markedly increases the frequency of tautomeric shift (chemical fluctuation due to movement of hydrogen atom from one position of purine or pyrimidine to another position) in 5 BU and it changes from its stable keto form (C=O) to its less stable enol form (COH). In its keto form it pairs with adenine but in its enol form it pairs with guanine thus inducing point mutation during replication.

Chemicals such as ethydium bromide, benzopyrene from smoke and acridine dyes can cause frameshift mutations in DNA.

When DNA polymerase copies the alter strand (alteration due to intercalating dyes), adding or deleting base pairs around the bulge formed by the bound mutagen causes the frameshift. (Snustad).

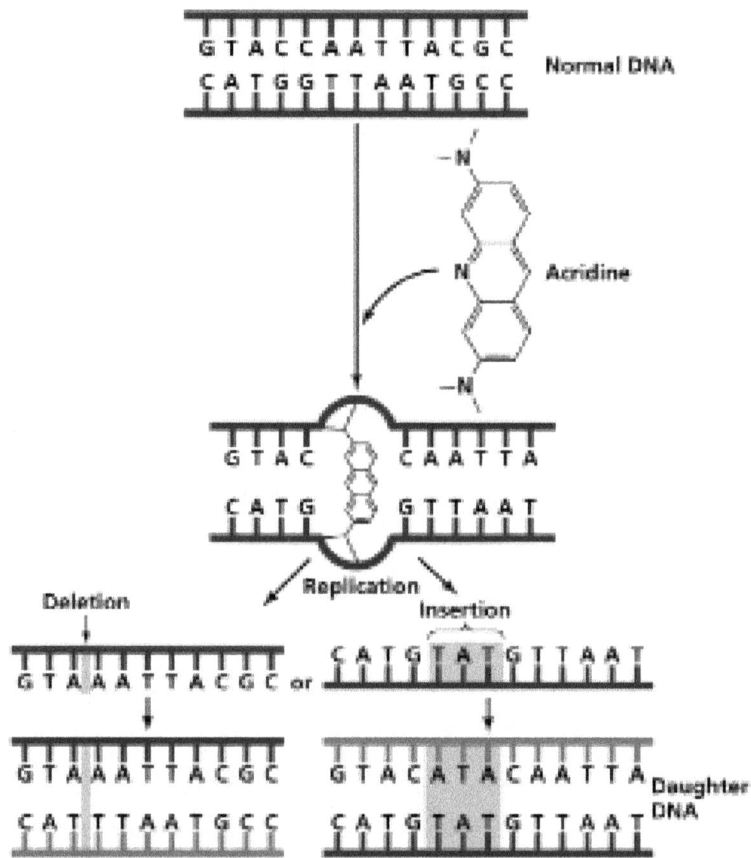

Procarcinogen The precursor of an active carcinogen. The procarcinogen itself is not usually carcinogenic but is converted to the active carcinogen after it has been metabolized. For example, the drug diethylstilboestrol (a synthetic oestrogen no longer in clinical use) is metabolized to an epoxide intermediate, which can cause cervical cancer.

Example: The pro-carcinogen benzo[a]pyrene, a major mutagen in cigarette smoke, becomes metabolized by the body's P450 system to produce a carcinogenic compound *i.e.* epoxide:

O_2, 2e⁻, 2H⁺ — CYP1A1 / CYP1B1 — H_2O

H_2O — Epoxide-Hydrolase

benzo[*a*]pyrene

(+)benzo[*a*]pyrene-7,8-epoxide

O_2, 2e⁻, 2H⁺ — CYP1A1 / CYP1B1 — H_2O

(-)benzo[*a*]pyrene-7,8-dihydrodiol

(+)benzo[*a*]pyrene-7,8-dihydrodiol-9,10-epoxide

Once formed, the carcinogen tends to intercalate into DNA (the aromatic region can Pi stack with the nitrogenous bases) and react at the epoxide region to form a covalent bond at guanines. This inclusion distorts the structure of DNA, causing errors in DNA replication (G - T transversion). If these mutations occur in a gene regulating the cell cycle, cancer may arise. (C.B. Powar)

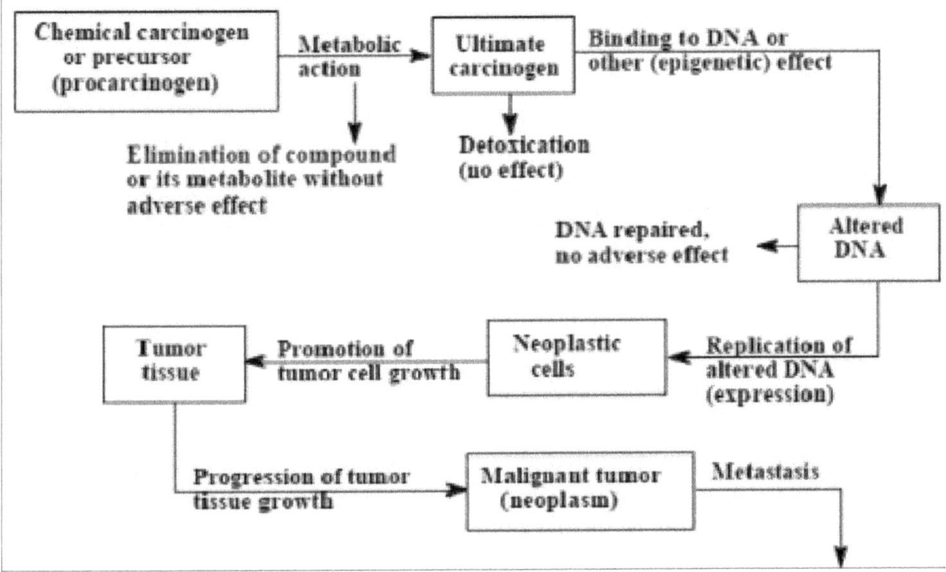

Cancer Therapies

(A) Radiation Therapy

Radiation therapy is the medical use of ionizing radiation as part of cancer treatment to control malignant cell growth. Radiotherapy can be used for curative or adjuvant cancer treatment. It is used as palliative treatment (where cure is not possible and the aim is for local disease control or symptomatic relief) or as therapeutic treatment (where the therapy has survival benefit and it can be curative). Total body irradiation (TBI) is a radiotherapy technique used to prepare the body to receive a bone marrow transplant.

Dose

The amount of radiation used in radiation therapy is measured in gray (Gy), and varies depending on the type and stage of cancer. For curative cases, the typical dose for a solid epithelial tumor ranges from 60 to 80 Gy, while lymphoma tumors are treated with 20 to 40 Gy.

Preventative (adjuvant) doses are typically around 45 - 60 Gy in 1.8 - 2 Gy fractions (for Breast, Head and Neck cancers respectively.) Other factors that are considered while selecting a dose include whether the patient is receiving chemotherapy, whether radiation therapy is being administered before or after surgery, and the degree of success of surgery. *(Baldock, 2010).*

Fractionation

The total radiation dose is fractionated (spread out over time) into smaller doses so that normal cells get time to recover, while the tumor cells are less efficient in repairing the damage between fractions and tends to undergo cell death. Fractionation also allows tumor cells that were in a relatively radio-resistant phase of the cell cycle during one treatment to cycle into a sensitive phase of the cycle before the next fraction is given. In USA, Australia, and Europe, the typical fractionation schedule for adults is 1.8 to 2 Gy per day, five days a week.

Tumors that regenerate more quickly when they are comparatively smaller in size have different treatment regimen. Two fractions per day are used for such tumors near the end course of treatment. This schedule, known as a concomitant boost regimen or hyperfractionation,

Example: Continuous Hyperfractionated Accelerated Radiotherapy (CHART) CHART, used to treat lung cancer, consists of three smaller fractions per day. *(Ang, K. Kian 1998).*

Mechanism of action

Radiation therapy leads to DNA damage of the cancer cells thus inducing apoptosis. The damage is caused by a photon, electron, proton, neutron, or ion beam directly or indirectly ionizing the atoms which make up the sugar phoaphate backbone of DNA helix. Indirect ionization is caused as a result of the ionization of water molecules, forming free radicals (hydroxyl radicals), that finally damages the DNA. Cancer cells are undifferentiated in nature and behave like a stem cell, they multiply in number, and have a diminished ability to repair sub-lethal damage (caused by radiation) compared to most healthy differentiated cells. The DNA damage is inherited through cell division, accumulating damage to the cancer cells, causing them to die or reproduce more slowly.

One of the major limitations of radiotherapy is that tumor cells in a hypoxic environment become resistant to radiation damage than those in a normal oxygen environment. Solid tumors can outgrow their blood supply, causing a low-oxygen state known as hypoxia. Oxygen is a potent radiosensitizer, increasing the effectiveness of a given dose of radiation by forming DNA-damaging free radicals. Thus in oxygen deficient environment they exhibit resistance.

Types of Radiation Therapy: The are three main divisions of radiotherapy are:

1. External beam radiotherapy (EBRT or XBRT) or teletherapy
2. Brachytherapy or sealed source radiotherapy
3. Systemic radioisotope therapy or unsealed source radiotherapy.

The differences relate to the position of the radiation source; external is outside the body, brachytherapy uses sealed radioactive sources placed in the area under treatment, and systemic radioisotopes are given by infusion or oral ingestion.

1. External beam Radiotherapy
   a) Conventional external beam radiation therapy or 2-Dimentional radiotherapy
   b) 3-Dimensional Conformal Radiotherapy (3DCRT)
   c) Intensity-Modulated Radiation Therapy (IMRT)
   d) Image-guided radiation therapy (IGRT) or four-dimensional radiotherapy
   e) Hadron Therapy
   f) Stereotactic Radiotherapy (Cyber Knife, Gamma Knife)
   g) Tomotherapy
2. Brachytherapy or sealed source radiotherapy
   a) Mold brachytherapy
   b) Strontium plaque
   c) Interstitial brachytherapy
   d) Intracavitary brachytherapy
   e) Intravascular brachytherapy
3. Unsealed source radiotherapy

External Beam Radiotherapy

(a) Conventional external beam radiotherapy: It uses linear accelerator machines to deliver two-dimensional beams. It consists of a single beam of radiation delivered to the target site (tumour) from several directions: front or back, and both sides. The term *Conventional* refers to the way the treatment is *planned* or *simulated* on a specially designed calibrated diagnostic x-ray machine known as a simulator. The simulator recreates the linear accelerator actions to a well-established arrangement of the radiation beams to achieve a desired *plan*. The aim of simulation is to accurately target or localize the volume which is to be treated. The limitation of this therapy is that high dose radiation may lead to damage of the healthy tissues surrounding the tumor volume which in turn can cause secondary neoplasm.

(b) **An enhancement of virtual simulation is 3-Dimensional Conformal Radiotherapy (3DCRT)**, in which the profile of each radiation beam is shaped in such a way that it fit the profile of the target (tumour) from a beam's eye view (BEV) using a multileaf collimator (MLC) and a variable number of beams. Since the treatment volume conforms to the shape of the tumour, the relative toxicity of radiation to the surrounding normal tissues is reduced. Thus this technique allows a higher dose of radiation to be delivered to the tumor than conventional techniques.

(c) **Intensity-Modulated Radiation Therapy (IMRT)** is an advanced type of high-precision radiation. IMRT conform the treatment volume to concave tumor shapes which are associated to vulnerable structures, such as tumor wrapped around spinal cord or a major organ or blood vessel. Computer-controlled x-ray accelerators distribute precise radiation doses to malignant tumors or specific areas within the tumor. The pattern of radiation delivery is determined using programmed computing applications to perform optimization and treatment simulation (Treatment Planning). The radiation dose is consistent with the 3-D shape of the tumor by controlling or modulating the radiation beam's intensity. The radiation dose intensity is elevated near the gross tumor volume while radiation among the neighbouring normal tissue is decreased thus elimination radiation toxicity.

(d) **Image guided radiation therapy (IGRT)** or four-dimensional radiotherapy allows locating the tumor under the linear accelerator just before the irradiation, by direct visualization (3D mode soft tissue) or indirect visualization (2D mode and radio-opaque markers). The technical implementation of IGRT is done by complex devices. (Lagrange JL; 2010).

(e) **In particle therapy** (Proton therapy), energetic ionizing particles (protons or carbon ions) are directed at the target (tumor). In case of heavier particles dose increases while the particle penetrates the tissue and gradually loses its energy. Dose increases up to a maximum (the Bragg peak) that occurs near the end of the particle's range, and it then drops to (almost) zero. The advantage of this energy deposition profile is that less energy is deposited into the healthy tissue surrounding the target tissue.

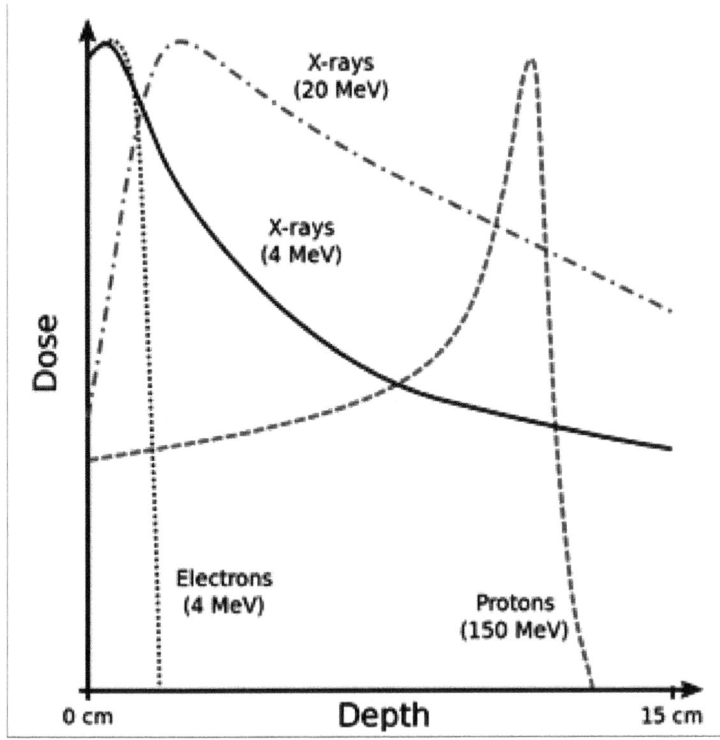

(f) **Stereotactic Radiotherapy** is a type of external beam radiotherapy that focuses high doses of radiation within the body, with high accuracy. Cyberknife and Gamma Knife are the current technologies.

- **Cyberknife:** The two main elements of the Cyberknife are (1) the radiation is produced from a small linear particle accelerator (2) a robotic arm which will allow the energy to be directed at any part of the body from any direction thus increasing its accuracy.

6D Skull

The X-ray camera images are compared to a library of computer generated images of the patient anatomy. Digitally Reconstructed Radiographs and a computer algorithm determines on the motion corrections that need to be given to the robot because of patient movement. This imaging system allows the Cyberknife to deliver radiation with an accuracy of 0.5mm without using mechanical clamps attached to the patient's skull thus making it non-invasive. This technique is commonly known as *frameless* stereotactic radiosurgery. This method is referred to as 6D because corrections are made for the 3 translational motions (X, Y and Z) and three rotational motions.

- Gamma Knife contains 201 cobalt-60 sources of approximately 30 curies (1.1 TBq), each placed in a circular array in a heavily shielded assembly. The device aims gamma radiation through a target point in the patient's brain. A specialized helmet is surgically fixed to the skull of the patient, so that the brain tumor remains stationary at the target point of the gamma rays. An ablative dose of radiation is thereby sent through the tumor in one treatment session, while surrounding brain tissues are relatively spared. Gamma Knife radiosurgery accurately focus many beams of gamma radiation to converge on one or more tumors. Each individual beam is of relatively low intensity, so the radiation has little effect on intervening brain tissue and is concentrated only at the tumor itself where all radiation converges.

(g) **Tomotherapy** is a type of radiation therapy in which the radiation is delivered slice-by-slice. Its precise radiation beams are continuously produced to treat inoperable tumours. The inbuilt CT scanning helps in confirming the size and position of the tumour prior the treatment.

Brachytherapy or Sealed Source Radiotherapy

Brachytherapy uses temporary or permanent placement of radioactive sources. The temporary sources are usually placed by a technique called afterloading. In afterloading a hollow tube or applicator is surgically implanted in the organ to be treated followed by loading it with radioactive sources.

- **Mold brachytherapy,** Superficial tumours can be treated using sealed sources placed close to the skin.

  Method of inserting radon seeds (sealed radiation source) into a carcinoma of the lower lip, each seed was pushed through the embedding needle and into the tissue, where it was left permanently

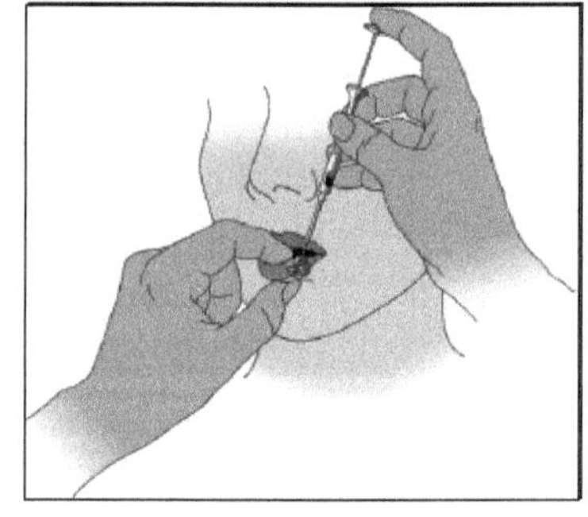

- **Strontium plaque,** used for very superficial lesions less than 1 mm thick. The plaque is a hollow, thin silver casing that encloses a radioactive strontium-90 powdered salt. The beta (electron) particles produced from strontium's radioactive decay have a very shallow penetration.
- **Interstitial brachytherapy**. The sources are inserted into tissue. Low Dose Rate prostate brachytherapy treats prostate cancer by using iodine-125 or palladium-103 seeds. The radioactive seed is placed into the prostate gland. Prostate gland is located close to the bladder and rectum, it is important for radiation treatment to be tightly focused on the prostate to avoid serious side effects.
- **Intracavitary brachytherapy** places the sources inside a pre-existing body cavity. Example: Delivery device may be inserted into a body cavity such as the vagina or uterus or into nasopharynx (upper part of throat behind the nose)
- **Intravascular brachytherapy** places a catheter inside the vasculature through which sources are sent and returned.

Unsealed Source Radiotherapy

Unsealed source radiotherapy relates to the use of soluble forms of radioactive substances which are administered to the body by injection or ingestion. These radioactive substances are typically used for their biological properties, which are similar to their non-radioactive parent substance.

Iodine is an element selectively taken up by the thyroid gland in healthy people as it is a vital component of the hormone produced by the gland. In papillary thyroid cancer radioactive iodine (iodine-131) is used which through natural uptake get concentrated into the thyroid gland. Iodine-131 produces beta and gamma radiation. The beta radiation released destroys thyroid cancer that takes up iodine whilst most of the gamma radiation escapes the patient's body. Most of the iodine not taken up by thyroid tissue is excreted through the kidneys into the urine.

(B) Chemotherapy

Chemotherapy is a category of cancer treatment that uses cytotoxic drugs to kill cancer cells. This results in the most common side-effects of chemotherapy: myelosuppression (decreased production of blood cells, hence also immunosuppression), mucositis (inflammation of the lining of the digestive tract), and alopecia (hair loss).

Dosage

The standard method of determining chemotherapy dosage is based on calculated body surface area (BSA). The BSA is usually calculated with a mathematical formula or a nomogram, using a patient's weight and height, rather than by direct measurement of body mass.

Types of Chemotherapeutic Agent

(a) **Alkylating agents:** They bind covalently to DNA via their alkyl group. DNA is made of two strands and the alkylating agent may either bind twice to one strand of DNA (intrastrand crosslink) or may bind once to both strands (interstrand crosslink). When the cell tries to replicate cross-linked DNA during cell division, or tries to repair it, the DNA strands break. This leads programmed cell death called apoptosis. Alkylating agents work at any phase of the cell cycle and thus are known as cell cycle-independent drugs.

(b) **Antimetabolites:** Anti-metabolites are a group of molecules that impede DNA and RNA synthesis. They have similar structure to that of DNA and RNA. The nucleotides comprises of a nucleobase, a sugar and a phosphate group. The nucleobases are divided into purines (guanine and adenine) and pyrimidines (cytosine, thymine and uracil). Anti-metabolites resemble either nucleobases or nucleosides (a nucleotide without the phosphate group), but have altered chemical groups. These drugs either block the enzymes required for DNA synthesis or get incorporated into DNA or RNA. Inhibiting the enzymes activity (involved in DNA synthesis), prevent mitosis as the DNA cannot replicate itself.

Misincorporation of the molecules into DNA displaces the double helix thus inducing programmed cell death (apoptosis). Unlike alkylating agents, anti-metabolites are cell cycle dependent. They only work during S-phase (the DNA synthesis phase).

(c) **Antifolates:** These analogues are antagonistic to folic acid, and block the function of folate-requiring enzymes. Folic acid is crucial for DNA metabolism. Antifolates could suppress proliferation of malignant cells, and could thereby re-establish normal bone-marrow function.

The anti-folates include methotrexate and pemetrexed. Methotrexate inhibits dihydrofolate reductase (DHFR), an enzyme that synthesizes tetrahydrofolate from dihydrofolate. When the enzyme is inhibited by methotrexate, the cellular levels of folate coenzymes diminish which are required for thymidylate and purine production, essential for DNA synthesis and cell division.

(d) **Fluoropyrimidines:** The common examples of fluoropyrimidines are fluorouracil and capecitabine. Fluorouracil is a nucleobase analogue that is metabolised in cells to form active products; 5-fluourouridine monophosphate (FUMP) and 5-fluoro-2′-deoxyuridine 5′-phosphate (fdUMP). FUMP becomes incorporated into RNA and fdUMP inhibits the enzyme thymidylate synthase; both of which lead to programmed cell death or apoptosis. Capecitabine is a prodrug of 5-fluorouracil that is broken down in cells to produce the active drug.

(e) **Anti-microtubule agents:** Anti-microtubule agents are plant-derived chemicals that block cell division by preventing microtubule function (polymerization and depolymerisation). Microtubules composed of two proteins; α-tubulin and β-tubulin. They are hollow rod shaped structures that are required for cell division. Vinca alkaloids and taxanes are the two main groups of anti-microtubule agents. These groups of drugs cause microtubule dysfunction but their mechanisms of action are completely opposite. The vinca alkaloids prevent the formation of the microtubules (polymerization). Taxanes prevent microtubule disassembly (depolymerisation). Thus they prevent the cancer cells from completing mitosis leading to cell cycle arrest finally inducing programmed cell death (apoptosis). These drugs can affect blood vessel growth (angiogenesis).

The **vinca alkaloids** (vincristine and vinblastine) bind to the tubulin molecules in S-phase and prevent proper microtubule formation required for M-phase *i.e.* prevent spindle fibre formation.

Taxanes (paclitaxel) promote microtubule stability, preventing their disassembly (prevent separation of chromosomes during anaphase). Paclitaxel prevents the cell cycle at the boundary of G2-M.

(f) **Topoisomerase inhibitors:** Topoisomerase inhibitors are drugs that affect the activity of two enzymes: topoisomerase I and topoisomerase II. When the DNA double-strand helix is unwound, during DNA replication or transcription, the adjacent unopened DNA winds tighter (supercoils). The stress caused by this effect is sustained by the topoisomerase enzymes. They produce single- or double-strand breaks into DNA, reducing the tension in the DNA strand. This allows the normal unwinding of DNA to occur during replication or transcription. Inhibition of topoisomerase I or II interferes with both of these processes.

Combination Chemotherapy

Cancer cells become resistant to a single agent, thus by using different drugs *concurrently* would help to overcome resistance to the combination.

(*i*) Methotrexate (an antifolate), vincristine (a Vinca alkaloid), 6-mercaptopurine (6-MP) and prednisone — together referred to as the POMP regimen —induced long-term remissions in children with acute lymphoblastic leukaemia (ALL).

(*ii*) Nitrogen mustard, vincristine, procarbazine and prednisone — known as the MOPP regimen —cure patients with Hodgkin's and non-Hodgkin's lymphoma.

Resistance to Chemotherapy

Resistance is a major cause of treatment failure in chemotherapy one of them is the presence of small pumps on the surface of cancer cells that actively move chemotherapeutic drugs from inside the cell to the outside. Cancer cells produce high amounts of these pumps, known as p-glycoprotein, in order to protect themselves from chemotherapeutics.

Drug Delivery

Most chemotherapy is delivered intravenously, although a number of agents can be **administered orally** (*e.g.*, melphalan, busulfan, capecitabine).

There are many **intravenous methods of drug delivery**, known as vascular access devices. These include the winged infusion device, peripheral cannula, midline catheter, peripherally inserted central catheter (PICC), central venous catheter and implantable port. These devices have different applications regarding duration of chemotherapy treatment, method of delivery and types of chemotherapeutic agent.

Targeted Therapies

Specially targeted delivery vehicles aim to increase effective levels of chemotherapy for tumor cells while reducing effective levels for other healthy cells thus resulting in an increased tumor kill and reduced toxicity.

Nanoparticles

Nanoparticles are 1-1000 nanometer (nm) sized particles that can promote tumor selectivity and can deliver low-soluble drugs. Nanoparticles can be targeted either passively or actively. Passive targeting exploits the difference between tumor blood vessels and normal blood vessels. Blood vessels in tumors are "leaky" because they have gaps from 200-2000 nm, which allow nanoparticles to escape into the tumor. Active targeting uses biological molecules (antibodies, proteins, DNA and receptor-ligands) to target the nanoparticles to the tumor cells. There are many types of nanoparticle delivery systems which include silica, polymers, liposomes and magnetic particles. Nanoparticles made of magnetic material are used to concentrate agents at tumor sites using an externally applied magnetic field.

Minicells

The minicells are derived from mutated bacteria. In these mutant strains, the cell division septum is aberrantly placed adjacent to the cell pole instead of at its normal midcell site. The polar septation events give rise to spherical cells (minicells) that lack the bacterial chromosome (no nucleus) but otherwise appear normal. These cell are loaded with chemotherapeutic drugs and coated with antibodies that target specific tumor cells. The 400-nm-wide spheres are large enough to be contained by normal blood vessels but small enough to slip out of the leaky vessels found inside tumors.

Monoclonal Antibodies

Monoclonal antibodies are targeted to tumor antigens expressed by malignant cells.

(C) Hormone Therapy in Cancer

Cancer arising from certain tissues including the mammary gland and prostate gland may be inhibited or stimulated by appropriate changes in hormone balance

(*i*) Prostate cancer is often sensitive to finasteride, an agent that blocks the peripheral conversion of testosterone to di-hydrotestosterone

(*ii*) Breast cancer cells often highly express the estrogen/progesterone receptor. Inhibiting the production (with aromtase inhibitors) or action (with tamoxifen) of these hormones can often be used as an adjunct to therapy.

(D) Immunotoxins for Targeted Cancer Therapy

Immunotoxins target the surface of cancer cells by using protein toxins capable of killing a cell with a single molecule. These potent proteins include plant toxins like ricin, saporin, and pokeweed antiviral protein (PAP), which inactivate ribosomes; and single-chain bacterial toxins such as diphtheria toxin (DT) and Pseudomonas exotoxin (PE), which inhibit protein synthesis by adenosine diphosphate (ADP) ribosylating elongation factor 2. (Robert J. Kreitman; 2006)

Mechanism of Action of Plant Toxins

Plant holotoxins (class II ribosome inactivating proteins) include ricin, abrin, mistletoe lectin, and modeccin. Hemitoxins, or class I ribosome-inactivating proteins, include PAP, saporin, bryodin 1, bouganin, and gelonin. Holotoxins contain both binding and catalytic domains, whereas hemitoxins contain only catalytic domains. Plant toxins prevent the association of elongation factor-1 and -2 (EF-1and EF-2) with the 60s ribosomal subunit by removing the base of A 4324 in 28s rRNA and Ricin also removes the neighboring base G 4323 thus inducing apoptosis. Only the enzymatic domain of both holo- and hemitoxins translocates to the cytosol. The binding domains of holotoxins are removed by reduction of disulfide bond prior to translocation. The intracellular transport of ricin is dependent on sorting receptors that cycle between the endoplasmic reticulum (ER) and the terminal compartments of the Golgi. Glycolipids that bind ricin may be transported from endosomes to the Golgi. Lysine-aspartic acid-glutamic acid-Leucine (KDEL) ER retention sequence enhances delivery of ricin to the cytosol. (Robert J. Kreitman; 2006)

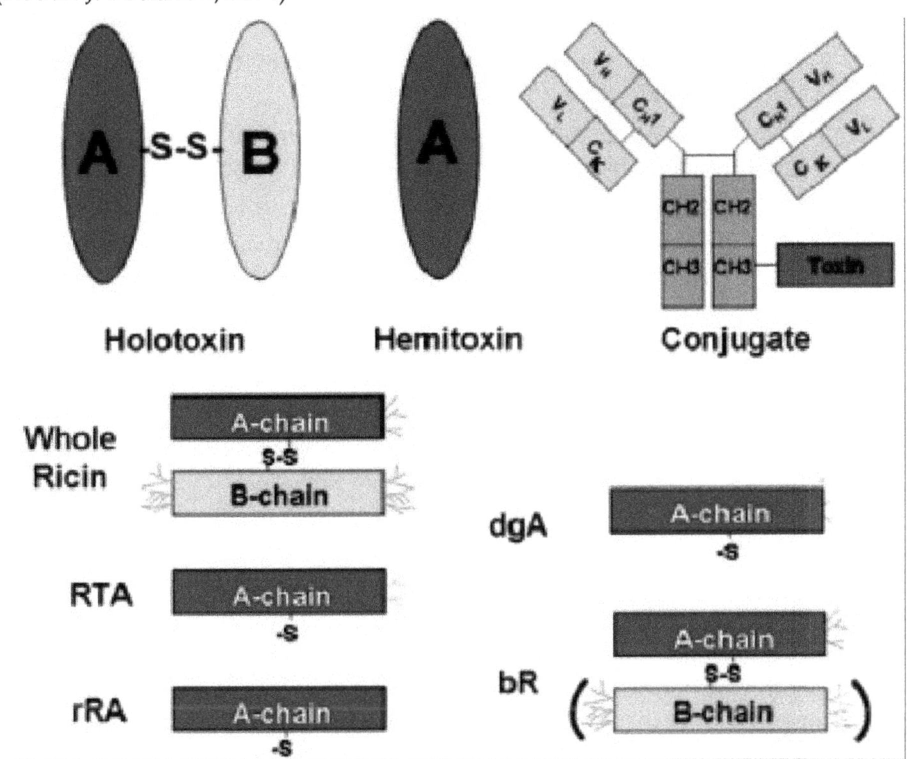

Mechanism of Action of Bacterial Toxins

Bacterial toxins (PE and DT) enzymatically ADP-ribosylate EF-2 in the cytosol. They each catalyze the ADP-ribosylation of histidine-699 of EF-2, which is post-translationally modified to a diphthimide residue. (Robert J. Kreitman; 2006)

Mechanism of Intoxication of PE

PE, is a single-chain protein (613-amino-acid) which contain 3 functional domains. Domain Ia (amino acids 1-252) is the binding domain, domain II (amino acids 253-364) is responsible for translocating the toxin to the cytosol, and domain III (amino acids 400-613) contains the ADP-ribosylating enzyme that inactivates EF-2 in the cytosol. The catalytic process of ADP ribosylation utilizes the following residues His440 and Glu553. His440 binds nicotinamide adenine dinucleotide (NAD) via Adenosine monophosphate (AMP) ribose. The carboxyl group of the Glu553 side chain, through a water mediated hydrogen bond with Tyr481 and Glu546, which allows Tyr481 to bind NAD through a ring-stacking mechanism.

Steps involved in targeting the toxin and killing the cancer cell:

(a) The C-terminal residue (Lys613) is removed by a carboxypeptidase in the plasma or culture medium.

(b) Domain Ia binds to the macroglobulin receptor that is present on animal cells and is internalized via endosomes to the transreticular Golgi.

(c) After internalization, the protease furin cleaves domain II between amino acids 279 and 280.

(d) The disulfide bond between cysteines 265 and 287, which joins the 2 fragments generated by proteolysis, is reduced.

(e) Amino acids 609 to 612 Arginine-glutamic acid-aspartic acid-leucine (REDL) bind to an intracellular sorting receptor that transports the 37 kDa carboxy terminal fragment from the transreticular Golgi apparatus to the ER.

(f) Amino acids 280 to 313 mediate translocation of the toxin to the cytosol.

(g) The ADP-ribosylating enzyme within amino acids 400 to 602 inactivates EF-2 thus inhibiting protein synthesis.

Inhibition of protein synthesis is sufficient to induce cell death by apoptosis. (Robert J. Kreitman; 2006)

(E) Gene Therapy in Cancer

Gene therapy is used to create recombinant cancer vaccines which trains the patient's immune system to recognize the cancer cells by presenting it with highly antigenic and immunostimulatory cellular debris. Initially cancer cells are harvested from the patient (autologous cells) or from established cancer cell lines (allogeneic) and then are grown in vitro. These cells are then engineered to be more recognizable to the immune system by the addition of one or more genes, which are often cytokine genes that produce pro-inflammatory immune stimulating molecules, or highly antigenic protein genes. These altered cells are grown in vitro and killed, and the cellular contents are incorporated into a vaccine (Deanna Cross; 2006).

References

Ana Maria Abreu Velez and Michael S. Howard; Tumor-suppressor Genes, Cell Cycle Regulatory Checkpoints, and the Skin, N Am *J Med Sci*. 2015 May; 7(5): 176–188.

Ang, K. Kian (October 1998). "Altered fractionation trials in head and neck cancer". Seminars in Radiation Oncology. **8** *(4): 230–236.* doi:10.1016/S1053-4296(98)80020-9

Baldock C, De Deene Y, Doran S, Ibbott G, Jirasek A, Lepage M, McAuley KB, Oldham M, Schreiner LJ (2010). "Polymer gel dosimetry". *Physics in Medicine and Biology.* **55** *(5): R1.* doi:10.1088/0031-9155/55/5/r01. PMC 3031873 PMID 20150687

C.B.Powar; Molecular Genetics of Cancer; Himalaya Publishing house

Deanna Cross, James K. Burmester, Gene Therapy for Cancer Treatment:Past, Present and Future; C linical Medicine & Research, Volume 4, Number 3: 218-227 ©2006 Marshfield Clinic.

H. Dertinger and H. Jung, "Molecular Radiation Biology", Springer-Verlag, New York, 1969.

http://mattjacksonblogger.blogspot.in/2014/10/uv-light-and-mutation.html.

Lagrange JL, de Crevoisier R, [Image guided radiation therapy (IGRT)]. Bull Cancer. 2010 Jul;97(7):857-65. doi: 10.1684/bdc.2010.1140.

Lawrence A. Loeb, Keith R. Loeb, and Jon P. Anderson; Multiple mutations and cancer; Proc Natl Acad Sci U S A. 2003 Feb 4; 100(3): 776–781.

M. Iwamoto, D. J. Ahnen, W. A. Franklin, and T. H. Maltzman, *Carcinogenesis,* 21,1935–1940 (2000).

Rastogi RP, Richa, Kumar A, Tyagi MB, Sinha RP; Molecular mechanisms of ultraviolet radiation-induced DNA damage and repair. *J Nucleic Acids.* 2010 Dec 16;2010:592980. doi: 10.4061/2010/592980.

Robert J. Kreitman; Immunotoxins for Targeted Cancer Therapy; *The AAPS Journal* 2006; 8 (3) Article 63 (http://www.aapsj.org).

Santarosa M, Ashworth A: Haploinsufficiency for tumour suppressor genes: when you don't need to go all the way. *Biochim Biophys Acta* 2004; 1654:105.

Snustad & Simmons; Principal of Genetics. 8th Edition; *John Wiley & Sons.* 2006.

Zhang W, *et al.,* MicroRNAs in tumorigenesis: a primer. *Am J Pathol* 2007; 171:728.

Innovations in Biochemical Techniques (2020) : Page no. 175-
ASTRAL INTERNATIONAL (P) LTD., New Delhi - 110002

Index

D

D

F

G

H

I

L

M

www.ingramcontent.com/pod-product-compliance
Ingram Content Group UK Ltd.
Pitfield, Milton Keynes, MK11 3LW, UK
UKHW021011290726
14059UKWH00001BA/73

9 789390 371624